CW01511305

Published in Great Britain by

L.R. Price Publications Ltd., 2022.
27 Old Gloucester Street,
London,
WC1N 3AX
www.lrpricepublications.com

ISBN-13: 9781915330390

JON'S STORY
A STRANGER TO MYSELF

A Personal Reflection
on Mental Health

Jon Conroy

This book is dedicated to all those who have or who continue to suffer with mental health issues or childhood trauma.

PREFACE

My name is Jon and you don't know me. After all, why should you? So I find myself writing a book on my own mental health and people ask me, 'Why?'. Well first and foremost, I guess, I have a story to tell but who doesn't? Yet I feel compelled and I don't think that's too strong a word, to share my story with others. If I'm honest, there have been people who have tried to persuade me that this is not the right course of action and part of me gets that but I have a stronger desire and that is simply to help others. You see, my primary aim in writing this book is to help anyone out there who is crying, alone, in the darkness of his or her own life.

Right from the start, however, I want to make something abundantly clear - that if you are suffering from any kind of mental health trauma then please seek professional help as soon as you can. You see, I am just an ordinary guy and I have no professional qualifications in this area at all but I do have something and that is, a story of a life to tell and that is what I want to share. For this reason, at its heart is the fact that the very essence of this book is that it is nothing more than a personal reflection. Hence all I am inviting you to do is to join me on a journey that will take us into the darkness but eventually, we will emerge together out into the light. At times you may well find some of the things I have to say deeply upsetting but this cannot detract from their truth and perhaps, the need for them to be shared.

In all honesty I have tried to be, throughout the pages of this book, a person of integrity, decency and sincerity; something I hope which really comes through. My great hope is that there is someone out there who will read it and simply come to the conclusion, 'This helped me'. If just one person could say that, then I would be able to sit back and say to myself, 'Jon, that was a job well done'.

CONTENTS

Introduction   1

Part One - Exorcising the Ghost   7
Who Are You? - Chapter One   7
Getting Inside My Own Head - Chapter Two   14
I Can't Find Myself - Chapter Three   19
Learning to Surf - Chapter Four   24
Lessons Learnt - Chapter Five   33
Awareness - Chapter Six   39
So Is Everything About Me Then? - Chapter Seven   46
Breaking The Chains - Chapter Eight   56
Learning To Let Go - Chapter Nine   64
Getting To Know Myself - Chapter Ten   70
Marching To The Beat Of The Drum - Chapter Eleven 76
'Don't Worry – Be Happy' - Chapter Twelve   81
Fear Is The Key - Chapter Thirteen   88
'My Feelings Matter!' - Chapter Fourteen   94
'On Your Marks, Get Set, Go!' - Chapter Fifteen   99

Part Two - The Sun and the Moon   105
'Rebel – Rebel' - Chapter Sixteen   106
'Don't look back in anger' - Chapter Seventeen   117
'Don't give up!' - Chapter Eighteen   153
'Sticks in the Mud' - Chapter Nineteen   171
Is This the End or Just the Beginning? - Chapter Twenty
                                                      179

INTRODUCTION

'Who are you?'

Good question and I am not really sure that I know the answer! And I find that strange to say, to admit even to myself but at the same time, I know it's true. Then I find myself asking, *'Is it only me that feels this way?'*

'Who are you?'

But what does a question like that even mean? If you are taking the time to read this, have you ever asked yourself the same question and if so, why? I don't want to feel alone in trying to answer this and I would feel better if we could try to find the answer together.

'Why?'

See, what do you mean by why? Oh and by the way am I allowed to ask questions? Yes of course I am but you know what? You, yes I mean you the mysterious questioner, are not going to give me the answers are you? So where can I expect to find them? Instinctively, I want to say that the answers are in me but buried so deep I can't find them but I know, somehow, for some unknown reason that nevertheless they are there.

Somehow that helps. To think and believe that the answers to all my questions are accessible to me if only I could find them, brings me a sense of consolation. No - not a sense, that's the wrong word – feeling, seems better, more appropriate somehow.

'Why?'

It's because my feelings hold the key to everything. And that's what I need to understand.

'Are you happy?'

And there's the big one! Am I happy? I'm not even sure I know what happiness means. Do I know dark moods? Yes. Are there times when I feel so low I don't even know what to do or where to turn? Yes. Do I know depression? Yes. Do I know sadness? Yes. Do I know self-loathing? Yes. Do I know heartache? Yes. Do I know loneliness? Yes. Are there times when I feel that life has no meaning or purpose? Yes. Do I have thoughts of suicide? Yes. But as for joy, happiness and fulfilment – I would have to say, *'I'm not even sure I know what they mean?'* Have you ever felt like that? I know I can't be the only one but all too often it feels just like that. Yet I feel that happiness is there, lying somewhere beneath the surface of my life. Is it my fault that it will not come out or have I buried it so deep within me that I can't touch it anymore? Did I ever truly know happiness in the first place or was it all an illusion? Perhaps there is something wrong with me – I feel that there is but I'm not sure what, if anything, can be done about it. Sometimes I just feel sad, lost, walking through life but not really experiencing anything other than the distractions I hope can, at least for a while, keep me sane. Does this make sense to you, the reader? Because if it does then we are on a journey together. A journey that I hope will provide some answers.

'So what are you going to do about it then?'

There's another big one! I know how I feel, I've just told you but what do I do about it? Now that, as they say, is the sixty-four million dollar question. My head, but more importantly my heart, tells me that the key to everything lies within me. Why? Well that's where my feelings are and it's those feelings that I need to come to terms with if I am ever going to make any progress. My own feelings that I need to understand, feelings which in all honesty, eventually gave rise to my own seeds of self-destruction. But I have a problem and it's a pretty big one. In fact it's huge! You see I've had these feelings for as long as I can remember. They are part of me, part of who I am and I am not sure what to do about them. Which means I need help. I don't feel it's wrong to say that but at the same time, I don't want to give the impression that I am ill because somehow that misses the point. So what do I do? Tell people I'm depressed and get medication! Well that's one solution but I'm looking for something else. I'm looking to be able to sort things out for myself but I know I can't do this alone. So I have two options. Firstly, to do nothing and carry on as before or secondly, to say, '*You know what, perhaps I do need a little bit of help after all*'. I don't think that option one is a viable one for me anymore so let's give option two a try but please, no platitudes!

'*Help*.'

Before we get started let me say a few things. Firstly, I am no expert but who is when it comes to life? Every individual is unique and should be treated as such. No two people ever have the same feelings nor experience anything in exactly the same way. Secondly, this is not a self-help book because I want to avoid any sense of the answers to people's problems about life, being found in the pages of this book. The answers, in my opinion, are to be found in life and the experience of life itself. So in reality, the answers are within us, it's just that sometimes we lose our way a little bit. Thirdly, nobody ever teaches us anything about life! There's no school curriculum, course or preparation for what life is or how it's to be experienced. Instead, we're expected to pick it up as we go along. Some people do and that's fine but most of us struggle to make any sense out of anything and all we do is end up surviving – at least most of the time. And then there are those who don't – survive that is! What about them? What happens to them? Who helps them?

So what then, is the intention of this book? Well merely to observe. I am going to make a number of observations about life and how we live it. Many of these will be based on my own experiences, which I offer in all humility. Now if you find anything that I say useful, fine. However, if you find nothing I say useful, well that's also fine. I invite you to accompany me on a journey through life about life. Now let's see what happens but please remember, everything you read in the pages of this book are my own thoughts, my own opinions and my own ideas. I don't expect you to agree with me but you might find my own personal reflections on my own mental health interesting and possibly even helpful.

PART ONE

'EXORCISING THE GHOST'

'Who are you?'

CHAPTER ONE

I'm going to start this chapter with the most basic and fundamental question of all, 'Who are you?'. However, I'm going to begin with a story and let me give you the reason for this. My intention in this book is never to tell you what to do. Instead, my approach will be to encourage you to reflect on your own life in the light of your own experiences. Incidentally, I'll be doing exactly the same. As a result, any conclusions you come to will be your own. Remember it's your life and your experiences. Take what you find useful but try to stick with it. Only then will you be able to make clear-minded judgments and decisions for yourself. But please remember that even when we explore a story, try to reflect on what it might mean for you. Here we go then.

A man once found an eagle's egg and wasn't quite sure what to do with it. So being well-intentioned and passing a farm, he popped it into the nest of a chicken and off he went. Sometime later the egg hatched along with several chicks and the young eagle grew up with them.

Throughout the whole of his life, the eagle did exactly what his fellow chickens did, thinking mistakenly of course, that he was just another chicken. So he scratched the ground for worms and insects. He did his best to cluck and clack and he would even thrash his wings and on occasion managed to fly a few feet into the air.

Now years went by and the young eagle grew old. Then one day he saw a magnificent bird flying in the air above him in a beautiful, cloudless sky. The bird glided in graceful majesty among the powerful wind currents, with scarcely a beat of its strong, golden wings.

Once again the old eagle looked up in absolute awe, turned to his neighbour and asked, "Who is that?"

"That's the eagle, the king of the birds," replied his neighbour. "He belongs to the sky, just as we chickens belong to the earth." So the eagle lived and died a chicken, for that is what he thought he was.

Right, so what did you think of the story? Simple enough but what's the point of it? Well, let's start with who you are in the story. Who do you identify with the most? Is it the eagle flying high up in the clouds, freely roaming the skies? Or is it the eagle on the ground, scratching the floor, clucking and clacking, thinking he's a chicken? Of course, maybe you identify with the chickens themselves, I'll leave that up to you. So where does that leave us? Well, I think of it like this and these, of course, are my own thoughts; you can come to your own conclusions. What if we are all really eagles thinking and behaving as if we are chickens? Now there's a thought but what do I mean by that? In the story, the eagle in the sky is described as *'the king of the birds'*. The fact that the eagle on the ground, who remember, thinks he's a chicken and so behaves like one, doesn't change the fact that he is, in reality, an eagle and also *'king of the birds'*, he just doesn't realise it, he doesn't get it! And so, he continues to live his life completely oblivious to his own greatness. *'Poor old eagle'* I hear you say. But wait a minute, what if I'm the eagle living on the ground thinking I'm a chicken. What do you say to that? What if I'm oblivious to my own greatness? And what's more, what if you are on the ground there with me thinking you're a chicken too, when in fact you too are an eagle? What happened to your greatness then? Right, so here is the issue and it's a pretty big one to start off with. I'm asking the question, **'Who am I?'**. And I'm inviting you to do the same. I also want to know more about that eagle. Who told him he was a chicken? Couldn't he see that he was different from the other birds? Why didn't he do something about it for himself? And then when he saw the eagle in the sky, why didn't he recognise himself and change? I like these questions but they become harder when I apply them to myself. See here's the issue as I see it. What if I am the eagle scratching around on the ground, not even aware of my own greatness? Whose fault is that, mine or someone else's? Was I born like that or did I become like that? Do I blame myself or do I blame someone else? Do you see where I am going with this? Right, now what happens when I become aware of the fact that I am the eagle scratching around on the ground? What happens when I become aware of the fact that I am, in fact, nothing less than '*king of the birds?*'. That I am, dare I say, this, '*Great!*'. What do I do now? What do you do now?

I have options. I could say, you know what, I'm happy as I am in ignorant bliss! But I know this is not true. Why? Because I'm not happy! Secondly and this is the big one, I could suddenly realise that the source of my unhappiness is the fact that I am not the person I thought I was! At this point, the easy option would be simply to run away and hide but you know what? I've come this far, so let's explore what else I could do.

I've called this book, *'A Stranger to Myself'*, simply because that's how I feel, at least some of the time. If you've ever felt like that then we're on the same wavelength. Yet if I am ever going to be *'happy'* I feel that I need to get to know that stranger. I need to see myself from the inside out and learn how to live. So my first step is to face up to life. That is how I feel at the moment, in fact that's how I've felt for as long as I can remember. I don't feel that I'm really living but I want to! I hope that makes sense. That means that I can't run away, I have to face up to how I feel and do something about it. So running away isn't an option anymore. Instead, I have to take responsibility for my own life. But first I have to ask myself a really big question and when I do, I invite you to join me. And here it is: *'Do I really want to be happy?'*. I'm going to stress the word *really* because that makes the question even more important. Of course, if the answer is *'yes!'*, then the next question has to be, *'Okay, so what are you going to do about it?'*.

First of all we need to get certain things straight and the most fundamental point is, never tell me to be happy. Never tell me just how lucky I am. Never offer me platitudes or little anecdotes about life. Why? Because they don't work or even if they do, they never last. Now don't get me wrong, I'm not questioning people's motives or desires to help people like us, I'm just being straight with you and telling you what doesn't work. Putting it simply, I don't need to be told things. I hear the words, I even understand them but they have no impact on me, no effect on me, they pass straight through me. What I do need is to be able to feel something, to experience it from the inside because only then will I begin to truly understand. In fact, here we have the very core of what I am trying to say, it's just that no one I've ever met has really understood and so what's the point?

Right, so now let's get back on track. Do I really want to be happy? Yes! So what am I going to do about it? Step one appears to be to get inside my own head, to take responsibility for myself and to try and see and understand what is really going on within me. So let's get back to that eagle scratching around on the ground with those chickens, so misguided and confused being something that he is not and recognising and accepting that I am, in fact, that bird.

Can I, however, be happy now or only unless something happens outside of me? Can I truly be at peace with myself? Is it possible to know the stranger that I am to myself? This is going to be hard but you know what, I'm going to give it a try. Want to join me?

GETTING INSIDE MY OWN HEAD
CHAPTER TWO

Okay, I'm going to take a long hard look at myself and ask the question, *'Do I really want to be happy?'*. But straight away you come back at me and say, *'Really, of course you want to be happy, everyone wants to be happy!'*. But you know things are not as simple as that. Maybe I'm used to being unhappy. I'm more comfortable being like that, it's who I am and people expect me to behave that way.

'Right, so we're back to being the eagle who thinks he's a chicken then?'

Well yes, I guess we are.

'But didn't you say that you're an eagle, not a chicken, don't you know that, don't you feel that? Get back to the question you want to answer, 'Are you happy?' Or are you happy being unhappy?'.

I feel like my life has and continues to be, some sort of act. I am not the person people think I am but I don't know who I am and that's why I am *a stranger to myself!*

'Wow! That sounds like pretty heavy stuff to me.'

Yes but at least I feel that we are getting to the point. I need to be able to see things clearly for what they are. To recognise what is real and what is important. Maybe even to stop pretending, stop putting on an act. You see the life I'm living doesn't seem real. It's as if the events happening to me are, in reality, happening to someone else and there's nothing I can do about it. The first step is for that eagle to see himself as an eagle when everyone treats him like a chicken. Do you see what I mean? I feel that deep inside of me is a person that nobody knows, not even me and it's that person that I need to find and it's that person that I need to be. Looking at that sad little bird scratching around on the ground, I recognise myself and with that, I am beginning to see through things, recognising things for what they really are. Can I accept them though? Can I drop the pretence? Can I say that there is someone inside of me trying to get out, the person who I really am? You see, the struggle and the pain often comes with what people expect me to be and do and it's simply not who I am but I'm afraid and it's simply easier to remain unhappy.

There's a line from a Bob Dylan song that, from time to time, pops into my head and it goes like this:

'Got to change my way of thinking'. However, I need to be very careful here because I know from experience that wanting to change is not enough. Do you think I really want to be like this, live like this? Do you? Yet wanting to change never helps, in fact it only leads to greater unhappiness as I become more and more increasingly dissatisfied with myself. Do you see the problem?

'Right, so what do you do?'

Do you mean, what do we do?

'Okay then, what do we do?'

Let's start with a simple question like, *'What do I really want?'*. Well what I really want is to have the courage to be me, just me. Not who other people think I am. Not what other people want me to be. Just plain, old, simple me. Yet although the question appears to be simple and it is, I just can't find the answer.

'Is that because you don't really know who you are?'

Yes, I'm *a stranger to myself.*

'So where do you begin?'

I don't feel that I can, or indeed should, force anything. I feel I need to begin to understand myself, know myself. At the same time, I know that I never want to live my life simply to fulfil other people's expectations of me. I've tried that and it's the road to misery. So I need to have the courage to be me. I need to know who I really am. So I'm going to try something and if you want to, perhaps you can try it with me too. I'm going to observe myself, watch myself. I'm going to try and get to know me!

'How's that going to work then?'

Well, it seems to me that the very first thing I need to do is to try and understand who I am. I am not seeking to change myself in any way at all because I don't believe that will work. Instead, I am going to take a long hard look at my life along the following lines:

What do I do?

Why do I do what I do?

What are my reactions to things, people and situations?

What are my moods?

What do I say and why?

Where do I go and why?

What are my motives?

What do I think of myself?

What do I think other people think of me?

Who do I like and don't like?

Now whatever happens when I do this, I am going to try and not judge myself. I am going to try and have no connection whatsoever with what is taking place. At the same time, I am not going to fix anything or interfere with anything because that's not the point of why I am doing this.

'*So why are you doing it then?*'

Simply because I want to understand myself first and to achieve this, I need to see what's going on inside my head. I need to see myself from the outside in and the inside out! If things are going to change and I am ever to discover what true happiness really is, then I need to be able to answer the question for myself. '*Who am I, really?*'

I CAN'T FIND MYSELF!

CHAPTER THREE

'Well, did you find out who you are?'

Yes and no.

'What does that mean?'

It means that the answer to your question is a little more complicated than I thought it would be.

'Go on.'

Okay, this is what I discovered and to be honest, it surprised me. The fact is I came to the conclusion that it feels like I am two people. Listen, I know, at least in my head, that I am one person but how I live and experience life feels like I am two, almost different, people and that's what's causing many of my problems.

'You'll have to explain that to me as, to be honest, I don't get it and I expect few people reading this would understand what you are saying either.'

I'll give it a go but these are my own thoughts and experiences and they might not make sense to anyone else, even though I hope they do. Deep down inside of me there is the person who I really am and who I really want to be. However, that person is buried so deep that I struggle, most of the time, to find him. All I know is I want to be, need to be, that person, if I am truly to be free and live. Yet I am afraid that person is dead. For now I am going to call that person the **'I'**.

The second person I am going to tell you about, I am going to call the **'Me'**. This person is the person I think I am inside my head. So the **'Me'** person are my thoughts, my reactions and my experiences of life but it is not the **'I'** and therefore, not the person who I really am, the true me, the real me. Right, so now here comes the problem and it's going to sound complicated so I will try to make it as simple as possible. When the **'I'**, the person who I really am, identifies with the **'Me'**, the person in my head, then that is when I suffer. That is when I am unhappy. That is when life is unbearable.

'**Why**?'

Because I am not being the person who I really am!

'***Can you explain this a little more please?***'

I'll try! But to do this I am attempting to explain what is going on inside my own head and it's not easy. Firstly, I would love to be the real me. That is what I want. That is what I need if I am ever going to be truly happy but there is something stopping me, preventing me from achieving this and it's been going on for as long as I can remember. You see, I feel I live most of my life as someone else, the person I refer to as the *'Me'*. This then becomes the second issue for me and is directly related to my unhappiness and the way in which I feel about life. You see the *'Me'* actually cares about what other people think about him. The *'Me'* clings to labels given to him by other people and when those labels are attacked or threatened, the result is suffering and inevitable unhappiness. You know, I actually sat down the other day and wrote a list of the labels that actually mean something to me and here they are:

Status

Job / role / function

Money / possessions / things

Career

Qualifications

Approval / disapproval

Perception

Having done this I came to a startling conclusion that these are all important to the person I call the *'Me'*. So when any of the above are threatened I suffer and so become unhappy.

For me this was a **'WOW'** moment because I am actually saying that I care about what other people think about me and worse than that, I am allowing this way of thinking to run my life. No wonder I am unhappy then.

'So what would you like to do about it?'

Drop every single label I attach to myself which attempts to define who I really am.

'What's stopping you from doing that then?'

In a word, **'FEAR!'**. I allow fear to dictate to me who I really am.

'Go on.'

Take success or failure. I am actually afraid that if I am not successful I'll lose everything I have. So I actually care whether other people think I'm successful or not.

'But isn't that just in your head?'

What do you mean?

'Well you said it yourself when you were talking about what other people thought about you, because they may not be thinking that at all!'

You're exactly right because that may not be the reality of the situation. In other words, what's going on inside my head may not, in fact, be linked to anything real and if it's not real then it's an illusion and if it's an illusion, I am suffering unnecessarily! Or putting it simply, I am the cause of my own misery because everything is, in fact, inside my own head!

'Can you come to any conclusions about this?'

I am the cause of my own suffering and my own unhappiness by allowing myself to be the person I know, deep down inside myself, I am not. Every time the real person who I am identifies with the **'Me'** person inside my head, I suffer because that is not who I really am. Somehow I have to break this cycle and find a way to be free and I need to do this for myself from the inside out. I need to see the reality of life for what it is and not run away and hide because I am afraid. That person locked deep down within me, the one I know is the real me but who I am too afraid to be is, in fact, kept in slavery by the person inside my head. Time for a prison break then!

LEARNING TO SURF

CHAPTER FOUR

'So go on, what are you, sorry we, going to do now?'

Do you remember the story of King Canute? He was the guy who wanted to prove that he was only a man and could not stop the waves of the sea coming in. One day, I found myself on the beach in Whitby, West Yorkshire, watching as the tide came in. I remember just standing there staring at the waves as they crashed against the rocks. Life felt a bit like that, sometimes; overwhelming. Living up to other people's expectations, trying to be something I was not, being unhappy and just miserable. And there was nothing, so it seemed, that I could do about it! Or was there?

'Go on.'

Well, I thought later, as I reflected on my thoughts that day, 'What about surfers?'. Somehow, often against all the odds, they manage to survive the waves because they surf over them. The waves are still there - they don't suddenly miraculously disappear but the surfer learns how to ride them, how to survive them. Could it be, I thought, that life was just like that –

learning how to survive the crushing blows of the waves?

'Isn't that easier said than done though?'

Yes, but you've got to start somewhere and remember, I'm trying to work this out for myself. No doctors, psychologists, psychiatrists, counsellors or medication just plain, old, simple me! So give me time and give me space, I need to think. I need to build my own surfboard – the surfboard of life, you might say.

'How are you going to start that though?'

First and foremost I have to be totally upfront and honest with myself. So I am going to start with all those negative *feelings* I have. Here are just a few of them:

Feeling gloomy

Feeling down

Caring about what other people think and say about me

Feeling angry at life

Feeling unhappy

Feeling trapped

Being unable to motivate myself

Feeling jealous about people who seem to be happier than me

Feeling crushed by life

Feeling inadequate

Feeling unworthy and no good

I think I'll stop at this point because I'm running the risk of writing, literally, an endless list. The point is, that I have all these negative feelings inside of me dominating who I am and can, very often, see no way out. I am, therefore, trapped in my own prison of misery! The question is, did I create this cage, these bars and these prison walls for myself and if I did, can I do anything about them? You see, these are my waves and they are crushing me; I am literally drowning beneath them and I desperately need help. The only problem is that there is no one coming to my aid, there is no lifeboat, no life jacket and certainly no life guard who will plunge beneath the waves and rescue me. No, I am completely alone!

'Now that doesn't sound good.'

It's not, but I had to start somewhere and identifying my negative feelings by being honest with myself seemed to be, somehow, right. I then began to do something else by asking myself a question, *'What do I do with these negative feelings?'* To me, they were as real as anything else in life but for some reason, I felt the need not only to understand them but also, to do something with them. Right, so the first thing I did was to say to myself, '*These feelings are real and they are inside of me, inside my head – fact, period!*' Then I made myself go back to something I'd said earlier. Do you remember when I said that sometimes I felt like I was two different people: the real me, which I called the **'I'** and the person whom I thought I had to be because of other people, that I called the **'Me?'**.

'*I do but your description sounded strange to me. The 'Me' was the person you thought you had to be which, as a result, made you unhappy?*'

Yes that's exactly right.

'*The 'I' was the real you, who you felt you wanted to be but couldn't; the person buried deep within yourself.*'

True.

'*Right, now I've got that straight you can go on.*'

Okay, so I began to link all those negative feelings I described above with the **'Me'** the person who I felt forced into being but who, ultimately, was responsible for all my unhappiness. This was, in fact, the person I did not want to be. Instead, I craved to be who I really am! We are now coming to a breakthrough moment and I need to explain things very carefully to myself. If

I don't, the whole thing might just fall apart. Could it be that the source of the whole problem, in one sense, actually lay with me?

'*What do you mean by that?*'

Remember the '*Me*', the person I am not but the person other people expect me to be? What happens if I actually become that person? Imagine that, living a lie and becoming the very person, deep down, you know that you are **NOT**! Here then, is the very source of my unhappiness but it doesn't end there. This is because just like a magnet, it is the '*Me*' which attracts all those negative feelings I described above to it. Now the more the '*Me*' person I become, the more negative I feel but the whole thing is a lie because I am **NOT** that person.

Then one day I suddenly realised something for the first time: the '*Me*' does not really exist! No, instead I've just allowed it to consume me to become me but in truth, it is not real!

'*So what are you saying then?*'

I'm saying that the biggest mistake I ever made was to allow myself to become something I never was – *a stranger!* More than that, the person I really am but was afraid to be also became *a stranger!* So in that sense, I actually became a '**Stranger to Myself**'!

'*Hence the title of the book?*'

Exactly!

'*So what did you do next?*'

Firstly, the moment I realised all of this was when my liberation began and I started to learn how to surf the waves of life. My false self – the '*Me*', attracted all of those negative feelings I described earlier! So I said to myself, *'I am not that person, I was never that person, I don't want to be that person, what's more I don't* have *to be that person. All I want to be is free. Free to be the person I really am.'* You see, the more I allowed myself to be identified with the '*Me*', then the unhappier I became; to the point that all those negative feelings and this '*Me*' person who I had allowed myself to become, were one and the same. So could it be true that if all those negative feelings were inseparable from this '*Me*' person, who in essence was not real, then the feelings themselves were not part of reality either. All of a sudden I began to realise that I had, literally, become my own negative feelings. I had allowed these corrupting and life-denying influences to dictate who I was and how I lived. Putting it simply,

I had become my own negative feelings and it was destroying me.

The moment I realised this, things began to change. The *stranger* I have so far called the **'Me'**, I now actually recognised. This was not who I really was, of course, only a corrupted version of me created by a life which had not encouraged or allowed me to be myself. It was like recognising a monster, in one sense; a creature that had emerged out of my own personality by attracting and feeding on all those negative feelings.

'So what did you do now?'

I had to learn how to surf those waves. So I said to myself, 'You *are not your negative feelings!'* In fact, such feelings have nothing to do with the real you at all! It was now I had to simply learn to let go of this person I called, the **'Me'**. Thinking about it now, what I am really saying is that in one sense, I didn't really have to do anything all.

'Was it all in your head then, is that what you're saying?'

I would have to say '*yes*' and '*no*' to that question. 'Yes' because all of this is in my head and 'no' because all of the feelings I have described so far, were real and had consequences both for others and myself. You see, what I'm trying to say is that I had to stop being afraid. The challenge was to find, or rediscover, the **'I'** that real me had locked so deep within myself, that he had become a *stranger* too. But if I could find him and embrace him, if I could learn to stop being afraid, if I could discover that happiness was possible, then those waves could be ridden and I could survive.

'Was this all about you then?'

Of course it was, it always had been. I needed to change. I couldn't be told that; it was something I had to discover for myself. Once I found that out, however, then something else dawned on me – big time!

'Go on.'

Reality does not change. Everything outside of me continued exactly the same as it had before. *'People are people,'* as they say, so they will still criticise you, put you down, demean and belittle you. Your job will still be your job, where you live will still be where you live and your friends will still be your friends. What has changed is you. And when you change, guess what? Everything changes. You see, it's not reality that needs to change but your perception of it. Up to this point you have allowed your false perception of reality to transform you into something you are not. When you change, all this dies and finally you can embrace, recognise and live the life you always craved.

When you ask me 'is this all about you?', I have to say, 'Yes!' I can't, and should never, try to change others but I can change myself. Don't get me wrong, it's a long and painful process but in the end I get to finally meet the *stranger* who is myself. I hope that this does not sound arrogant. I don't mean it to be, nor do I want to give the impression that I am obsessed with myself. Remember that this is just a personal reflection, which I am sharing with you, the reader. So to put things in a little more perspective, I made a startling discovery when I embarked on this journey and it is this: that if there is a problem with the world, then it is me. Yes me! Little old, insignificant me! Yet if I am the problem, perhaps I am also the solution but it is up to me and no one else, to do something about it.

LESSONS LEARNT

CHAPTER FIVE

One day I asked myself, '*What really matters in life? Is it what you do or who you are?*' Let's face it, very often many people, including me, define who we are by what we do. Think about it for a second and see if it applies to you. Unfortunately, here lies much of the problem because the minute we fall into this trap, we end up conforming to what other people expect of us and so live our lives accordingly. Then one day we wake up as somebody else and live our lives that way; happiness, peace of mind and contentment end up being thrown out of the window. So here's one of my first lessons learnt: have the courage to be yourself, be comfortable with yourself, spend time with yourself and dare I say it, be a law unto your own self!

'*Really*?'

Of course, think back to what I said a little earlier: you can't change other people but you can change yourself. In fact, you might be surprised that when you change, everything changes because you are seeing things, perceiving life, in a completely different way. No longer are you trapped into being someone else. No longer are you imprisoned, conforming to a life other people expect you to live. Instead you are living your own life by being you! When I say everything changes, I mean because you had all of those negative feelings attracted by your false self, that *stranger* who was living your life for you, is now, in fact, gone. What has emerged to replace it is nothing less than the real you and nobody can hurt that person anymore because you don't care what anybody else thinks about you, because you're free. Free to be yourself.

What this means, in effect, is that we now see the world and other people not as they are, but as we are or as I am. For me personally that was, literally, a '**WOW**' moment. For this reason I began to understand that I didn't have to try to make good things happen but rather, to allow them to take place. Then I began to notice something else about people and it is this: when you dare to be yourself or dare to be different, other people will be too. Then came another one of those '**WOW**' moments for me and it is this: '*No one, and I repeat no one, has the power to hurt you anymore!*' In the same way, '*no one has the power to put any kind of pressure on you either anymore.*'

Why, I hear you ask? *'Simply because you are free to be yourself and at that point, all blame just slowly melts away.'*

'At this point I'm tempted to say 'WOW' myself! Can you summarise this for us please? You know, give us some rules for surfing all by ourselves, so to speak?'

I can and I will but please remember I am merely sharing my own thoughts and experiences with you, the reader. I am not writing a guide or a self-help book. Having said that, I will gladly summarise and share what I have learnt so far. If you find what I have to say helpful then that can only be a good thing. On the other hand, if you don't find it helpful, well that's fine too.

Rules for Surfing the Waves of Life

1. **Identify all those negative and destructive feelings lurking within you.**
2. **Understand that they are within you and not in the world – they are not part of what might be called external reality.**
3. **Do not see them as an essential part of who you really are. They are feelings and the**

thing about feelings is that they come and they go; they will not be with you forever.

4. Understand that you, and only you, can do something about such feelings and that when you change, everything changes.

5. Understand that you are responsible for your own negative feelings because they live inside you, not anyone else.

6. You have no right to demand or have expectations of other people.

7. Never punish yourself for feeling negative. Instead, give yourself time, recognise them and accept them, then simply acknowledge that they will eventually pass.

8. Live your own life. Do NOT allow anyone else to have any kind of power over you.

9. Make sure that when you are making a decision, you are acting as a response to something rather reacting to your own negative feelings.

10. Stop trying to be something or someone else. Realise that the place you were being forced to go is not where you have to be. In

other words, do not push yourself somewhere but realise you are, in fact, already there.

'Any more thoughts on the story you shared with us about the chicken and the eagle?'

Yes, one or two in fact. Thinking back to that story, imagine spending the whole of your life being told that you are a chicken! So what happens? You end up believing you're a chicken and so you live your life as, yes, a chicken! But the truth is that we are all eagles and the minute you realise that, everything changes. However, it is you who has to believe it and it is you that has to change. Not other people, not other situations but you, or should I say, me. When that happens and you discover and have the courage to be the real you, then that's the day when, perhaps, for the first time in your life you actually start to live. How liberating is that?

'Do you want to add anything else?'

I feel like I'm on a roll so yes, I will.

When I say, *'Be yourself'* or, *'Have the courage to be the real you'*, I don't mean merely copy or imitate someone else. That would be, in fact, a recipe for disaster. Instead, it's all really about having the courage to be you, to be comfortable with yourself. I know it's not going to be easy but then again, what is in life? Remember you are not expecting other people or other situations to change because they won't. So I'll say it again and again and again, when you change everything changes. Have a go for yourself, try it and see what happens. After all, what have you got to lose?

AWARENESS

CHAPTER SIX

As I've grown older and I hope a little wiser, the one word I have come to appreciate more and more is *awareness*. I don't think I was ever encouraged, personally, to be *aware* enough though.

'What do you mean by that?'

Well, I think we can look at this in two ways. Firstly, I never really thought about being *aware* of myself, you know, as a person.

'What does that mean?'

Actually it's hard to put into words but I'll give it a try and if you are not sure, just ask – okay? Right, here goes then. What does being *aware* of myself mean to me? I would have to say it starts from within. My own feelings, my own thoughts, my own experiences, even my own perceptions. I'm not talking about self-obsession here. No, I'm talking about knowing myself. Remember what I said earlier about being a *stranger to myself*?

'Yes – that's also the title of this book isn't it?'

Exactly and these are some of the reasons why that title is so important to me. Nobody ever encourages you to be *aware* of yourself. Think about it. We are encouraged to be *aware*, at least in part, of our surroundings and, of course, the needs of others but what about me and what about you? What about our needs? This, for me, should be the starting point. You see, my own problems started when I lost who I was; the real me, in one sense, died! If that's going too far and I don't think it is because these are my thoughts and my feelings and nobody else's, then I should be able to say what I like – right?

'That's up to you.'

Putting it a different way, the real person, or should I say the real me, became so buried deep within me that yes, I actually became *a stranger to myself*. And what replaced it was the false me, the conditioned me, the person that everybody else wanted me to be. In other words I ended up living a lie. We know what happened next, don't we, because I've already described it but I'll say it again. I resented the person I became. No, that's not strong enough; I hated the person I became. My life was one of misery and unhappiness, attracting and feeding off all of those negative feelings we explored earlier. To me that was not life, to me that was not living, to me I had, literally, become a complete *stranger to myself*!

'So what happened next?'

I'm coming to that but I would have to say that this is where the key word of *awareness* comes in. You see, the starting point must be that we are *aware* that this is what is going on inside of ourselves. Only I can do that and I must do it for myself because nobody else can experience what I am experiencing. Nobody else can tell me how I feel. Nobody else can tell me what is going on inside of me. And as I've said time and time again, nobody else can tell me to change. Instead, I must do all of these things for myself but the starting point has to be with me realising that something must be done. It would be great if schools, parents, social workers and all other people involved in helping others could see this, get this and encourage this but in truth, my experience is that nobody has the time, experience or expertise to do it. What I'm saying here is that before the crisis strikes, preparation would help.

I don't like saying this but again these are my thoughts and my experiences of life but it feels, at times, like the whole of society has been conditioned to prey off each other. In such a system,,, the strong survive whilst the weak and damaged become casualties. But does it have to be this way? Of course not but I'm not going to explore the bigger picture here just little, old, insignificant me. So let's get back to *awareness* then. Only when you become *aware* of what's going on inside of you can things begin to change, can things start to get better and the key to everything is you, or should I say me. Well it's both actually!

Just one more thing before I move one. The second point I want to make about *awareness* is that which concerns others and the surroundings or environment in which we live. These, of course, are important but I am not going to explore them in the pages of this book. All I would say is this, and once again, this is only my own opinion but I would make the point that, the moment we become *self-aware,* the more we become sensitive to and therefore *aware* of the needs of both others and the world in which we live; the two go, inevitably, together. This, in fact, is a point I will make later in the book; that the movement from being obsessed with our own lives, to that of concern for others and the world around us is, in fact, a healthy one.

That said, I can now move on. Once you've started this process of *self-awareness* you get to know more and more about the real you and that *stranger* which had taken over your life begins to fade, albeit gradually, away, taking all those negative feelings about life with him. Now you learn to be at ease with yourself and, perhaps, crucially and most importantly, you start to drop all of those fears, which previously had held you back. Once lurking in the shadows of my life was the desperate need to be liked by others, to impress others, to be needed by others and to fit in with the expectations of others. If on the odd occasion the real me surfaced, then I found myself apologising or explaining, excusing even. Imagine that, making excuses and apologies for being me!

'All of this sounds terribly sad.'

Of course it does but your pity and sorrow won't help me. No! I must help myself. I must become *aware* as to who I really am. I must learn to live my own life, to be the real, authentic me and not to become a *stranger to myself.* Do you get this; do you understand what I am trying to say and why I am saying it?

'I think so but I want to know more.'

One day I thought to myself, does anybody really accept or reject you and by this, I mean the real you? Could it be that they are accepting or rejecting what they only think is you? After all, who really, and I mean really, knows you apart from yourself, that is? So could it be that people are accepting or rejecting only an image of you and an image which they, in fact, have created for themselves? So in reality, people are not accepting or rejecting you at all because the truth is that they don't even know you.

So I began to learn a life lesson and it is this. Have no expectations at all of others; equally, make no demands from others for your own well-being. Try to define happiness for yourself. Go on – give it a try and see what happens. I'll tell you what will happen, shall I? There is no such thing because your definition of happiness will, in all likelihood, be totally different to everybody else. The danger is that if I define happiness, I will attempt to impose it onto you and if, as a result, you are not happy, I may come to the conclusion that there is, in fact, something wrong with you. Do you see what I mean?

This then is what I mean by *awareness* but in particular *self-awareness*, in so far as the whole process starts with you or me. If you can see this, if in some way you get it, then it's, literally, like waking up. One day, I suddenly realised for myself that this whole process, this way of thinking, or putting it more accurately, this way of being meant one crucial thing and it is this: no one can ever hurt you again! No one can ever have any kind of power over you again! How liberating is that?

I'll end this chapter with a quotation from *Gandhi*, which when I first saw it made total sense in relation to everything I have tried to say so far.

'*Be the change you want to see in the world.*'

Wow, I thought, that's exactly it! It's not up to others but up to me. Only I have the power to change me. I can't change others but you know what, I can change myself and that change starts here and now!

SO IS EVERYTHING ABOUT ME THEN?
CHAPTER SEVEN

I think this is an important point to make so let me explain. The answer, putting it simply, is that it is and it isn't. You see it is, at least in one sense, all about me and I've made that point, consistently, all the way through the pages of this book so far. However, on the other hand it can't really be exclusively about me. This is how it works. When I become that *stranger to myself* and consequently absorbed all those negative thoughts and ideas, I ended up, inevitably, projecting them out of myself and onto other people. In other words, my unhappiness, whatever happiness means, will no doubt affect the happiness of others, especially those closest to me. But equally when I confront this *stranger*, challenge him and replace him with my true self, then the reverse happens. However, all of this depends on my own sense of *awareness* and the ability to discern what is actually going on inside my own head. Does that make sense?

'Yes it does but is there more?'

Yes there is. We've still got quite a way to go yet before I'm finished. Yet I feel I need to labour the point that I must change first because when I change, everything changes and therefore it's all down to me. You see, what I'm saying is that I'm not prepared to accept things the way they are. I am not prepared to die, in a mental health sense, in the blood of my own misery and unhappiness. Not when I'm prepared to do something about it. Not when I *can* do something about it. This is when I realised, perhaps for the first time in my life, that I am, in fact, empowered just by being alive, to act. To not accept things the way they are. After all why should I? After all why should you?

'So what's next then?'

You keep pushing me and challenging me, forcing me to put into words what, up until now, I've only ever thought about in my head.

'Can I stop you there and ask you another question?'

Go on.

'Why are you doing this? Writing this book I mean; after all you don't have to?'

I've obviously given that question a lot of thought because to be honest, I am not finding writing this book easy at all. In simple terms, I'm putting pen to paper in the hope that my experiences might, in some small way, help someone else. Even if one person reads these words and it helps them, the effort will be worth it but we shall see. How does that sound?

'Actually quite good but what's next then?'

I'm going to share another experience with you now, one that it took me a very long time to realise but when I did, it was one of those *eureka* moments! Let's go back to happiness, whatever that means by the way. Once I defined myself by my negative moods: pain, misery, suffering and self-pity to name but a few. But that's who I was and that's how I thought of myself. As a result, I was conditioned to live my life like that. Not all of the time, you understand, but when the black clouds descended, that was who I was, simple as that. You asked me earlier was it all about me? That's such a great question because when I felt like that, when I entered into a dark place, when the black clouds truly descended then it was, literally, all about me because there was no one else; there was nothing else. But, of course, the way you feel very often is expressed by the way you act, what we do and what we say and that, inevitably, impacts on others. Those who care about you ask, '*What's wrong, is there anything we can do to help?*' Whilst those who don't care learn, all too quickly, to avoid you. So in that sense it can never really be just about me. Having said that, it feels exactly like that at the time. You see, no matter how well intentioned people are, nobody else can really feel like me because in my opinion, that's just not possible. Can you see the mistake I was making though?

'I'm not sure I can. You'll need to explain it to me, slowly!'

The big mistake that I made, and I mentioned this earlier, was that I fell into the trap of defining my feelings with who *I* am. My feelings and indeed my moods may well be part of me but they are **NOT** me – I am **NOT** my feelings and I am **NOT** my moods! This for me was a major step forward because I suddenly realised that, as a fact, I was something other than that which I thought I was. I know that may well sound silly to some people but for me it was a *'eureka'* moment in my life.

'So what did it mean in a practical sense?'

Right now, don't get me wrong. In a practical sense there was no transformation overnight but there was the beginnings of a significant change in my life and a realisation that I could actually do something about how I lived, for myself. I did not have to accept things as they were. Do you know how that made me feel?

'*No.*'

Happy!

'*Tell me more.*'

Actually this is quite difficult to explain but I'll try. Once I told myself to stop associating who I am with my negative feelings, although I didn't realise it at the time, I was, in fact, confronting *the stranger* I had become. Putting it simply I was saying to him, '*I don't want to be you anymore, I want to be myself.*'! It was at this point that something else dawned on me. That up until now I had, in fact, a very low opinion of myself and I didn't realise how low my own sense of self-worth had become. In other words, I didn't like myself very much! Yet nobody I knew, nobody that was close to me, people who had known me all my life, would have known that. You see I didn't even know this truth myself. Here then was the root cause of many of my problems and the solution lay with me. So *step one* for me was to disconnect with all of my negative feelings because now I knew they were not me! *Step two* was to say to myself that my sense of self-worth was down to embracing who I really am and not what other people expected or wanted me to be. *Step three* was to come to the conclusion that my happiness, yes my own happiness, was not at all dependent on my feelings or my emotions.

'Okay, can I stop you there and ask for an example please?'

Right, let's take being disappointed. So I don't get a job I apply for or get the answer to a question completely wrong. I don't make the grade in something or my suggestion to a problem is laughed at. What happens? Of course I'm disappointed in myself, I've let myself down, I feel other people think badly of me, I'm an embarrassment, I want to run away and hide. Now, this is exactly the kind of thing I am talking about because I have identified who I am with my feelings, with my emotions and as a result, my whole mood changes and part of me wants to hit out, fight back and make someone pay! So what, then, does this say about me?

'That you're normal?'

Really and what's that supposed to mean? In fact, that's not a big help but I guess you're here to ask questions and help me explain what I mean. You know, when I sat down and thought about this, I summed everything up by concluding that because I had identified too much with my own disappointments in life, that was why I was, in fact, unhappy!

'There you go – normal!'

Normal – yes, but if you always feel like that, if your feelings and emotions dominate who you are to the point that you are living in a perpetual state of unhappiness, to me that's not normal.

'Right, I see what you mean. So what happens next?'

Once I've established to myself that I am not my emotions or my feelings, they may well be an important part of me but they will not define me. The next thing I have to do is recognise that feelings and emotions come and go. They are literally here today and gone tomorrow. In other words, they will pass and my happiness should not depend on them. This to me was another part of my liberation. By all means be disappointed but do not let that disappoint define who you are. In truth, you might be disappointed but other people may not be disappointed in you. Instead, because your feelings of self-worth are so low, you naturally feel that other people feel negatively about you because you feel that way about yourself. Hence you are basing your life on a false perception of others, which turns out to be a fallacy. The result, inevitably, is a life of misery but as I have said all the way through the pages of this book so far, it doesn't have to be that way.

When I realised this, it triggered off something else in the way I was thinking and behaving. How much of life is an illusion?

'I don't get what you are saying here. You will have to explain this a lot better.'

Very often, much of what I thought about myself was based on what I thought other people were thinking about me, but what if I was wrong? What if my whole perception of others was not true, that they were not, in fact, thinking about me like that at all? Now, if that was only partially true then it meant that much of the way in which I was living my life was based on a lie. How tragic is that for goodness' sake? In fact, you might even say how sad is that? My happiness, my sense of self-worth was based on what I thought other people were thinking about me which was, in fact, simply not true. Imagine that, living your life based on an illusion which had nothing to do with reality at all. This, then, brings me back to the point I made earlier that my resultant unhappiness here, then becomes directed outwards towards others. In that sense, living my life based on an illusion gave rise to me making my own unhappiness a reality, not just in my own life but in the lives of other people too.

'Right, so what's the key?'

We all fall into the trap, at least at some time in our lives, of thinking 'if I change my outside world, everything will be better'. Here's what I mean:

I'll go on a diet and lose weight

I'll join a gym

I'll change my image

I'll get a new job

I'll move house

I'll change my career

I'll be like someone else

I'll buy a new car

I'll apply for that promotion

The list, of course, is endless but you see what I mean? If I change the outside world, my inside world will improve and get better. I'll be a different person, I'll be a new man! Yet we know that this, for most people, just does not happen. This is because it is nothing more than an illusion. The change, as I've repeatedly said at least for me that is, must come from within first. In fact, I would say that change, the kind of change I've spoken about time and time again in the pages of this book, is essential to personal growth. It's just that most of us have become resistant to it. In many ways it's easier, far easier, to change the external world than it is to engage with what's going on inside our own heads. Yet how come so many film stars and rock stars, that appear to have everything, at least far as the external world is concerned, are so unhappy? Equally, and in the same way, why do so many people in the modern western world seek therapy? Finally, why are anxiety, depression, despair and mental health issues such a feature of our society today? One day I realised that this applied to me just as much as it applied to anyone else but I also appreciated something more. That it is our minds which, in fact, chains us or sets us free. For me, this would be the key to everything because by now. I was fully committed to no longer being *a stranger to myself.*

BREAKING THE CHAINS
CHAPTER EIGHT

Imagine you are trapped in another life. Think about what it must be like, waking up one day and thinking the life I'm living is not my own. How often have you heard a teenager say, '*I hate my life?*'. I never really understood how someone could actually feel like that, let alone say it, until now. That's why the title of this book, '*A Stranger To Myself*', means so much because it sums up for me, perfectly, how I felt. I was living another life, failing to be the real me, trying to live up to other people's expectations when all along, I was living, what I now call, an illusion. So I made a decision that this had to stop and to do that, I had to break the chains which had, for so long, kept me in captivity. Putting it another way, I had fallen into the trap of living a life in the *captivity of negativity*!

'*So what did you do?*'

The very first thing I had to do was stop and take a long hard look at myself to see what was happening to me. It didn't take me long to realise something very important and this is an issue I have already reflected upon in the earlier part of the book. I was actually giving power to other people to hurt me and this had to stop! Now this might sound a little complicated but I'll try my best to explain. Remember when I told you earlier that I was not living my life as my true self?

'Yes, that was the stranger you had become who was not the real you.'

Perfect – that's exactly right. Now, it was this *stranger* who was attracting all those negative feelings I told you about, which had the effect of making me desperately unhappy and miserable. It was at this point I had to realise, again, two very important things:

1. I was **NOT** that *stranger* but I had allowed him to consume the real me.
2. All of those negative feelings I described earlier may well have been based on a false perception by me of others who were not, in fact, thinking that way about me at all. Even if they were, why should I allow them to hurt me?

Yet again though, this was something I knew I had to do for myself; nobody else could do it for me. You might recall that I have used the term *illusion* quite a lot, so let me explain now what I mean by that. When I use the term *illusion* in the pages of this book, I am describing something, which at the time, I thought was real but in reality was not. For the most part, I associate this state of mind with the *stranger* or my false self.

'Can you give me an example which will help me understand things a little better?'

Take this book. Should I care if people read it or not? Equally, should I care if people like it or not? Now these are questions I am asking of myself but please be patient and you'll see where I am going. So, let's say very few people buy it to the point that sales are low. How might I respond to this? I could be extremely disappointed concluding that people don't like the book and therefore they don't like me. Such disappointment then leads to sadness, anxiety and unhappiness or in other words, my mood becomes one of extreme negativity and I'm trapped once again. But, on the other hand, could it be true that, perhaps, very few people actually know about my book and that those who have read it have, in fact, found it extremely helpful? If this was the case, then my previous feelings of negativity were based on a false perception of reality but I have let such feelings control me once again. Secondly, what about if the reception of the book is poor and that people do not like it after all? Here, once again, I fall into the pit of depression and despair. Now let's analyse this. First, I might ask the question, '*Who have you written this book for?*' The answer to that question is, as I've said all along, *myself.* Right, so you've done that, you've achieved that, the book is out there and you've helped yourself, right? Right. Secondly though, I've also written the book in the hope that by sharing my experiences with others it might help them. Therefore, it could be true that someone out that there has read this book and found it extremely helpful in relation to any mental health issues they might be experiencing; we just don't know. But we could conclude that if this is the case – job done! True? True! Now, the fact that some people out there might not like the book does not change this one little bit. Criticism, as you might say, goes with the territory.

See what happens when I change my negative feelings for my positive ones? See what happens when I stop, or prevent, that *stranger* dominating who I really am. See what happens when I refuse to become the prisoner of my own negative feelings? The result is liberation and freedom. I actually become free to be the person I really am. Yet the process to be truly healthy starts even before I write the book or seek to get it published because in many ways, everything begins with desire. If I seek a false sense of happiness, one out of tune with the real me, then I am on the road to disaster. So, my starting point always has to be with a refusal to cling to any sense of what I am going to call false happiness and boy, is that hard to do. We are surrounded with so much pressure telling us what happiness is; if only you had this, did that and wore this, then you would be happy. You have to speak in a certain way, behave in a certain way and look a certain way, all to conform to someone else's definition of happiness. The long-term effect of this is the corruption of our souls, of who we really are. We end up being afraid to be ourselves and often without even realising it, we become someone else. Yes, we become a *stranger* to ourselves.

But it really doesn't have to be this way. However, the answer lies with us and for me, one of the first steps was to recognise that such desire leads, first of all, to anxiety and ultimately to unhappiness. Remember earlier I used the term *'false happiness'*? By this I meant conforming our lives to the expectations of others in the hope that it will make us happy and it will, at least for a while but it won't last. Why? Because it's based on an illusion, something that is not, in fact, real and has nothing at all to do with the real you. Hence I would say refuse, point blank, to feed yourself with false thrills because they will only lead to a *false happiness* and you will end up living a lie and hence, eventually, become a *stranger* to yourself. I know this because it happened to me. It took a while for me to work these things out but in the end I did and on that day, I found something precious – the truth!

You see I realised something - that no one could help me find this truth; I had to discover it for myself. To do that, however, I had to drop every single illusion I had about myself along with what I thought other people were thinking about me. When this happened, I was beginning to take my first steps on the road to true happiness because for the first time in my life, I was making true contact with reality.

'Wow, do you need a break?'

Not just yet. Let me explain something else first then I'll finish this chapter. For a long time in my life I was hypercritical of myself, to the point that I believed that nothing I ever said or did was good enough. In fact if I'm totally honest, part of me still feels like that to this day, even in writing the pages of this book! You see, I have to tell the truth otherwise there's no point in embarking on a project such as this. As a result, I found it relatively easy to condemn myself, literally all the time! However, by going through the process I have outlined in this book so far, I gradually began to appreciate and understand something and this might surprise you because the person I did not understand was myself!

'You're right, I am surprised and so I have to ask why?'

If you think about it, the answer is obvious. I had become a *stranger to myself*! So, once again, I took a good, hard and long look at myself and asked, '*What are you reacting to and why? What is making you think and act like this? Why are you so unhappy all of the time?*' Then something else struck me and I realised, once again, the **TRUTH** and it was this. That for the whole of my life I had been afraid and if we are not very careful, we always end up hating what we fear. In many ways it was like a fog or a cloud which had been covering me all of my life and preventing me from being who I really am. It was at this point I had to learn something very important, in fact, crucial if I was to make any kind of further progress.

'What was that?'

I had to learn to let go.

'Of what?'

Of everything!

LEARNING TO LET GO
CHAPTER NINE

When I sat down to write this book, the first thing I had to do was to try and bring all of my scattered thoughts together but little did I know how big a job this would be. For a start, how far back in time would I have to go? When did I first become aware I was thinking like this and finally, could I even do it? As I've already said, the key word '*awareness*' would play, for me, a major role in the whole process because it was only when I became *self-aware*, that I could begin to do anything about it. So when I asked myself, '*How far back do you have to go?*', the answer was, '*It's up to you. Just say what you need to say and leave the rest up to the reader.*'

I've already mentioned another of my key words and that is '*fear*'. When I thought about it, it was remarkable as to how much I had let '*fear*' dominate my life and how '*fear*' had actually prevented me from being my real self. When I put '*fear*', craving and desire together it was like confronting *ghosts* who had haunted me all my life and I had happily, allowed them to do so. You see, in this book I am not going to play the blame game. You won't find me blaming other people at all. Instead you will find only me, standing alone in the darkness. I must *exorcise these ghosts* for myself and to do that, I must confront reality as it is and not as I have wrongly perceived it.

'*That sounds really deep to me.*'

In one sense it is but I have to start off by saying that the key to making any kind of progress, is convincing myself not to be afraid and that's not going to be easy.

'Why?'

Because I've been afraid all of my life!

'*So where are you going to start?*'

One day I discovered something and I needed time to think things through, to see whether what I had been mulling over was, as a matter of fact, anywhere near the truth. To get to the bottom of this I'll start with a question. '*Are we programmed in life to need things?*' Notice I'm not saying 'by someone' but I'm asking the question in a more general way. Here's an example. Take success. Are we programmed to crave success? If we are, at least theoretically, some of us and here I mean me by the way, become afraid of failure. The same applies to acceptance, approval and appreciation, all of which are linked to success. So if I want to be accepted, gain the approval of others and be appreciated then I must be successful and if I'm not, well you know the answer to that one.

Now let's take it a stage further. When I was young I was under the impression that to be happy you must, and here we go:

- have money
- be successful
- have a partner
- get a good job
- have deep and meaningful friendships
- own your own house
- have qualifications

I could go on but you can see what I mean. Here I was being presented with a set of criteria for happiness. So the key to a happy and successful life was aiming for and possessing, all or some of these things. It felt like, even though I never realised it at the time, that I was being spoon-fed my happiness for life recipe.

'So what did you do?'

What most people do, I went for it! Imagine spending your life fighting to survive to achieve *the happiness list*, which will have the effect of, you guessed it, making you happy. The only problem is that one day you wake up and you find it doesn't. They can provide what I might call distractions or temporary thrills but they will, in and of themselves, not make you happy. Well that's my opinion anyway. What's more, you also find out something else, that bit-by-bit, little by little you start to lose your true self. The person who you really are, slowly and surely, begins to die or at least becomes so buried deep within you that you can't find him or recognise him anymore. Then the real truth hits you and it hits you hard. One day you look into the mirror and you don't recognise the person staring back at you because you've become a *stranger to yourself.*

   'That sounds terrible.'

It is and it isn't because the breakthrough comes when you are *aware* of what's happened because then, and only then, can you let go. Up until this point you have, in one sense, been living another life as another person but things can change and the key is *learning to let go.*

I got to the point, then, whereby I had to learn, literally, to let go of all those things, which were telling me, '*This is what will make you happy*'! At this point, I was beginning to feel that only by doing that would I really know what real happiness for me might mean. You see, in one sense, I had built my own prison and for the first time in my life, I was actually able to see the bars. It was at this point that I realised that I had, in fact, the power within myself to break free and fly. And this brings us back to that story I shared with you at the beginning. Do remember it?

'*The Chicken and the Eagle?*'

Yes – that's the one. You see for all those years, I had lived my life thinking and believing I was a chicken.

'*How so?*'

Well, I began to see, perhaps for the first time in my life, that I'd been fed on a diet of false happiness, whereby other people had told me what I needed to be and do if I was to be truly happy. That, of course, gave birth to this new person, the one I had become, *the stranger to myself* but I would be that person no more!

You know it sounds strange now as I write these words down but one day I must have said to myself, '*I'm going to stop being afraid. I'm going to let go of all those things I thought I needed to be and do to be happy! I'm going to stop allowing other people to have power over me. Instead, I'm going to be the real me.'* When I realised this, perhaps for the first time in my life, I actually felt free.

GETTING TO KNOW MYSELF
CHAPTER TEN

I've always maintained, throughout the pages of this book, that it is not a manual or a guide for self-help so please don't think it is or treat it as such. All I'm trying to do is share my own thoughts with the reader in the hope that you might find them interesting or helpful in some small way. The reason why I'm saying this again, is to make the point that nothing in this book is simply about '*trying harder*'. You see, it's been my experience that the more you resist something then the more it has power over you. It's like building the bars of your own prison cell. I've already made the key point that the breakthrough for me happened when I simply became *aware* of what was happening to me. My next step was to try to understand it. Therefore, imagine waking up one day and thinking, '*You're too afraid to live*'! Wow! But, and here's the thing, you don't have to do anything!

'*I don't get it!*'

Right, remember that *stranger to myself* I had become?

'*The one tied to all that unhappiness?*'

That's the one! Well he wasn't real! I had just allowed him to be. So if that was the case, all I had to do was let go. The mad thing was that for so long, I had just lived that life to the point whereby it had become reality for me. But the day I let go, the day I became *aware*, the day I realised reality was something different I was just seeing it in the wrong way, then that was the day when everything began to change.

You see, there's all the difference in the world between reality and how we see reality. Sadly, when we see reality in the wrong way and end up living our lives that way, the result is wasted time! So I took a good, hard look, at myself and said, '*You don't have to live your life like this anymore*'. Now remember, I've already made the point that it's not about change, it's about letting go. Then gradually, what began to emerge over time was the real me. When I began to see the world differently, that was the day when everything changed. Then I had another '*eureka*' moment!

'Go on!'

I didn't have to change! I didn't have to do anything! Why? I hear you say. Because I was already there, it's just that I had never realised it before. All I had to do was live!

However, *awareness* like that doesn't just happen overnight. You might realise it or feel it but for it to actually become you takes time. One of the lessons I learnt very early on was that the harder you try to change, the worse it gets. That's why I prefer the term '*letting go*'. Equally, the more you try to resist something, the more power it seems to have over you. In that way, the *stranger* you have become grows stronger as his corresponding negative feelings increase. So the advice I gave purely to myself was, '*Stop fighting it! Just let go and see what happens*'.

One of the first lessons I had to learn was how to be alone with myself. That is, my true self. Indeed, that's exactly why I have called this chapter, **'Getting to know myself'**. It's actually much harder than it sounds because we are so used to, or should I say conditioned to, craving the company of others to the point that we need it and therefore we can't do without it, that we lose the ability to be alone with ourselves. Now don't get me wrong, being with other people is a natural part of our humanity but being comfortable with yourself in the company of others, now that's something completely different.

'You'll need to unpack that a bit more for me please.'

Okay, most of us in the company of others are conditioned to behave in a certain way, whether we realise it or not. However, and remember that I'm only talking about myself here!, part of me has always been afraid to be the real me in the company of others, especially people I don't know. So in that sense, I was never really free because my life was literally dominated by feelings of anxiety, worry and fear.

'Why, for goodness sake?'

I guess it was because I was concerned about how I thought other people perceived me, in so far as I never saw myself as good enough. It's as simple as that.

'So what did you do about it?'

I became *aware* of it. You see, I asked myself a number of questions such as:

'What if you're wrong?'

'What if people are not thinking about you in that way at all?'

'Why should it matter to you what people are thinking about you in any case?'

'Why are you allowing your life to be dominated by fear?'

'Would it be so bad if you simply let go and be yourself?'

None of this was easy because no matter what I say here about myself and my own feelings, I think we all know that we do actually care about what others think about us. It is also true to say that we convince ourselves that we care about what we *think* other people are *thinking* about us and how crazy is that?

I saw and recognised all of these characteristics in myself and that is what I mean about becoming *self-aware*. So I challenged myself to be alone with myself so that I could get to know the real me but to my great surprise, I found myself resisting! This was because, for as long as I could remember, I had allowed myself to behave and respond like this; to allow this *stranger* to dominate my life - but no more.

Then I recognised something; that the more I tried to get to know myself, the more I recognised trends which actively prevented me from making progress, such as how angry I was with myself and how disappointed. What I needed was *self-insight* but years of inbuilt conditioning were erupting, giving rise to inner turmoil. Or putting it another way, the *stranger* I had become was fighting with the *stranger* I needed to be. So what I needed, in fact, was to be able to heal myself or reconcile who I was with the real me. Yet all the time as I tried to do this, I felt consumed by negativity but the truth that kept me sane was that at least I knew, or at least thought I knew, what was going on. Then came a massive breakthrough!

'*I'm listening.*'

I thought about it and all those negative feelings I was having about myself:

- Self-condemnation
- Self-hatred
- Self-dissatisfaction

And I realised something. Something so mind-blowingly obvious that it had been staring me in the face all along; that the reality is, much of the damage done to us in life we do to ourselves. That's why pain from the past can hurt us so much and that's why my own false perception of reality, including what I thought other people were thinking about me, did me so much damage. Once I began to realise this, my days of captivity were over.

MARCHING TO THE BEAT OF THE DRUM
CHAPTER ELEVEN

This is going to be a summary chapter because I feel the need to revisit some of what I have said so far, by setting it out and explaining it in a different way.

'*Interesting title for the chapter though.*'

A little patience, my friend, and all will be revealed. However, I was interested to try and find out how come I had never seen any of this before. So before I start, please remember, and I know I keep saying this but it's important to me, that these are purely my own thoughts, observations and comments. Once again, if you find them helpful that's fine but equally, if you do not find them helpful at all, that's fine too.

It just struck me that such negative ways of thinking and looking at life had been engrained in me from a very early age. Now I'm not saying that this was, in any way, intentional and that somebody sat down one day and said, '*Right, let's treat people like this*'. What I am saying, however, is that on reflection, it was like I had been conditioned to act and respond to life in a certain way. So if I go back to my earliest memories it was as if I had been encouraged to seek, almost as a measurement of my own happiness:

- *approval*
- *attention*
- *success*
- *status*
- *prestige*
- *acknowledgement*

Now of course, if you expect, want or need such things in life because you have been encouraged to do so, then what happens if you either do not achieve them or if you do, dread losing them? Putting it simply, my answer to this question is we, or rather more accurately I, hated the thought of:

- *failure*
- *making mistakes*
- *getting things wrong*
- *losing control*
- *any kind of criticism*

As a result and as I said earlier, we end up building the bars of our own prison cells. I could also say that living like that meant that my life was dominated by fear. In this way, I was giving power over how I lived my own life to other people and the result for me, was to live a life of misery. Of course, I was not *aware* of this at the time but my life became increasingly tuned into the reaction of others, which meant that I actually cared what other people thought of me. Imagine that - not living your own life but living your life based on what you *think* other people *think* about you. That, my friend, is the reason why I have called this summary chapter: **'Marching To The Beat Of The Drum'**, because it sums up for me, perfectly, a life lived based purely on the approval of others. Putting it another way, my happiness was a conditioned response to the approval or disapproval of others. Now what kind of life is that?

'Right, so what did you do next?'

Well, it provoked me into asking certain questions such as:

'Why do we need the approval of others so much to make us happy?'

'Why do we constantly need other people's encouragement and reassurance?'

'Why are we so dependent on what we think other people expect us to be and do?'

'Why are we so afraid to truly be ourselves?'

'What prevents us from seeing and realising the truth behind all of this?'

After all, nobody teaches us any of this because everyone is so busy conforming to the expectations placed on all of us, all the time, by others. So the more I thought and acted in this way, the more I became conditioned to seeing and accepting it as reality. After all, what else was there?

So you asked me, *'What I did next?'* The answer is I had to realise, first of all, that everything I have said so far was true. Secondly, I also had to appreciate that only I could do something about it and that therefore, I was the key to my own happiness. Not somebody else but me. The solution, if you like, was in my own hands or more accurately, in my own head. I call this process of realisation *'awareness'* or more accurately *'self-awareness'*. The day when you realise for the first time that you can be free, that you do not have to let other people have any kind of power over you, is truly liberating. You see, that's the day when you suddenly realise that you've been living a lie, that you've been living your life as someone else, as a slave to the expectations of others or putting it another way, as a *stranger*. Once this happens, you can start to rediscover who you really are and stop being afraid to be your true self. Then, perhaps, for the first time in your life, you can leap into the air and discover that you - yes you - can fly. As a result, you can leave the chicken behind because your destiny has been revealed. You are, in fact, an eagle.

'*I want to shout hurray!*'

Don't let me stop you my friend, so let's say it together!

'*HURRAY!*'

'DON'T WORRY – BE HAPPY'

CHAPTER TWELVE

There's an old Irish saying that goes, '*Worry is like a rocking horse and it gets you nowhere!*' Imagine that though, wasting all that time and all those years worrying about what you *thought* other people *were thinking* about you, only to find out that none of it might have been true! Imagine spending all that time seeking the approval and recognition of others, chasing success and status, only to discover that it did not lead to the happiness you were led to believe it would. All that worry and all that stress and it's got you absolutely nowhere! Although in one sense it has because finally you have become truly *aware* of everything and have begun to see reality in a completely different way. The eagle has finally taken to the air and a new life has begun. How exciting is that!

I've always found that there are plenty of people who will tell you to be happy but very few encourage us to find happiness for ourselves. You see, the simple truth is that nobody, I repeat nobody, really knows what's going on inside of me apart from me. As I've repeatedly said throughout the pages of this book so far, I might be the problem but I'm also the solution.

'So come on then, what did you do after you became aware of all of this?'

Having told myself it's perfectly okay to be me, to be, in fact, who I really am and not some *stranger to myself,* the first thing I needed to do was to, literally, let go of everything and drop the lot. All the hang-ups, the need to be wanted, the desire to be successful, to live life according to other peoples' expectations, you know all that stuff I've already mentioned; simply to let it all go. So I told myself, *'Just be who you really are'.* It was at this point that I suddenly realised something else, that I had actually forgotten how to enjoy myself. I'd been so conditioned to live according to the expectations of other people, that I had lost touch with what really made me happy. How mad does that sound? You see, I'd wasted so much time on what I thought would make me happy that I'd craved the same stimulus over and over again, not realising that I was stuck in an endless cycle. In the end, I came to the conclusion that none of these so-called 'things' would ever make me really happy. That's I why I had to continue, constantly, to replace them. Imagine treating people like that? That is, treating people like commodities as a means to an end. No, that's not how I wanted to live my life and I said to myself, *'Enough is enough'*.

How many times did I actually say to myself, *'I've not got enough time!'*? When what I really meant was, *'There's no time to really enjoy life'*. As a result, I would often find myself guilty of *'self-condemnation'*, always on the go, always feeling guilty, never quite achieving what I thought I wanted to achieve. So my first step to free myself from this never-ending cycle of misery was a simple one, to slow down. Sometimes people talk about 'the simple pleasures of life', but what are they?

'What, you mean you really needed to ask that question of yourself?'

Why don't you answer it then?

'Ah, now that's not my role in this book, so it's back over to you my friend.'

Right so, I asked myself, *'When was the last time you really tasted something or smelt something or even listened to something to the point where you could actually say, I really enjoyed that?'* I know that might sound sad to many people but what's the point of writing this book if I can't be honest with myself? Now here's the thing, I was conscious of, not so much, changing myself because that's not the best way to explain what was going on, but rather of allowing things to happen, if that makes sense. I mean, how many times do we hear people but not really listen to them? The solution to this isn't to change myself but to allow myself to actually listen to something that is already taking place, which might be a conversation with someone for example. What about seeing a flower or a bird or anything for that matter? We know it's there but do we really see it? It's that real feeling of enjoyment that I had to, somehow, recapture.

   'What do you mean recapture?'

   Because I associate the kind of enjoyment I'm talking about with aspects of my childhood, like jumping in a puddle or throwing a stick in a stream, eating ice cream and playing football, all because you simply love it. When you've got enjoyment like that, you suddenly realise and appreciate that, in fact, you need very little.

   'Aren't you just trying to go back and relive your childhood though?'

Absolutely not! I am, though, trying to apply to my life now what I learnt then. That happiness isn't something that you're fed by someone else, a sort of second-hand happiness. Rather, it's something only you can experience for yourself. To achieve this you don't have to change yourself at all but simply allow the experience to happen through you.

I appreciate that much of what I'm trying to explain in this book might be hard for some people to comprehend. That's why, as far as I am concerned, knowledge by itself is never enough. Rather, you have to taste and experience for yourself the truth of what I'm trying to say here. There is all the difference in the world between knowing something in your head and feeling it in your heart. The first does not always lead to change but the latter can lead to the transformation of your life. In other words, you don't have to force anything, you don't have to push against the flow at all; instead, the key is just allowing things to happen, naturally. This is something I again refer to as *awareness,* which for me changed and continues to change everything.

In the midst of all of this, I learnt something else: the need to be both honest and open with myself. Up to this point I had seen life as being hard and tough, the survival of the fittest if you like but I realised that this was not the kind of life I wanted to live and what's more, I didn't have to because it was up to me. So what's wrong with being gentle, kind, open and generous? Hence I discovered a subtleness to all of this, alongside the need to be flexible and open-minded. It takes great courage to do what I decided was needed next and that was to let all that negativity, typified by the criticism and judgement of others and all that unnecessary worry, stress and anxiety to pass straight through me. When that happened I decided that nothing like that would ever control me, have power over me or hurt me ever again. What I am describing here, then, is nothing less than a genuine moment of *self-discovery*. The key was to stop worrying, just drop it and let it fall away and to say to myself, *'It's all right to be happy because at last you are free!'* I know that I am describing something very personal and it might be hard for you, the reader, to understand but I am doing the best I can to record my own personal insights here.

Imagine then if you will, what it must be like to discover for the first time in your life that it is perfectly all right to be happy. Not somebody else's version of happiness but something you have discovered for yourself, to the point that it's not theoretical anymore because you can actually feel and experience it. That for me was, and continues to be, a genuinely **WOW** moment! Hence I could literally say, or should I say sing to myself, '*Don't worry, be happy*'!

FEAR IS THE KEY

CHAPTER THIRTEEN

I remember once hearing or reading, I can't remember which, that *'there is nothing in life to fear except fear itself'*. How true that is, but once again it's not enough to know the words, you have to experience them or live them. In other words, this phrase has to be lived if it is to become a reality in your life.

'I take it you're going to explain that?'

I'll certainly give it a try my friend. Once again however, this is something you have to discover for yourself. As a result I would make the following claims:

- **Fear** *prevents* us from doing what we want to do
- **Fear** *prevents* us from being our true selves
- **Fear** *prevents* us from really living
- **Fear** *prevents* us from being truly *aware*

Following on from this this I would then add that **fear** can lead to a wasted life because it's based on:

- *anxiety*
- *worry*

- *stress*
- *burdens*
- *concerns*

This might seem obvious to say but life is meant to be lived and it took me a long time, personally, to get things in perspective. But as I began to appreciate this fundamental truth about life, that's when things began to change.

'So go on, tell us, what did you do next?'

To answer that, I'm going to provide you with a little summary of what I discovered, personally, I needed to do if my life was to be changed and I was to become my true self. I'm going to call it here, letting go of **fear** and this is a short list of my findings:

1. Drop any and all illusions you might have and try to see and experience life as it really is. Remember that any perceptions that you might have about other people and what you think they might be thinking about you, are probably wrong.

2. Make every effort to let go of any kind of dependency because the fear of losing something or someone will only haunt you.

3. Learn to be alone! Try it and see how difficult it is for any length of time.
4. Recognise that in reality, other people do not have any power over you at all. Therefore, the truth is, no one has the power to make you happy or miserable.
5. Learn to see life in a new and different way as if you're doing so for the first time.
6. Refuse to need anything!
7. Make a promise to yourself: *'I will not fear anything or anyone anymore!'*
8. Try your best not to crave any kind of appreciation.
9. Learn to be at peace with yourself.
10. Be strong enough to say, *'Life does not have to be this way!'*

'Is that it?'

You're funny you are and no that's not it, not yet anyway. You see, there was something else I discovered and it was crucial to any kind of progress I wanted to make. **Fear** is negative and I have reflected on the impact negativity had on my life and with it, the *'stranger to myself'* I had become as a result. So the key for me to make any kind of progress was to replace the negative way I had been thinking with something far more positive. This meant that I to learn some new skills, many of which did not come easy and would require a lot of practice. So here we go with yet another list!

a) I had to try to learn the skill of patience in an infinite sense.

b) To think positively given any situation.

c) To enjoy things I had previously found difficult, such as work, but for the right reasons.

d) To learn to laugh again and to enjoy the company of other people.

e) To appreciate enjoying and doing things which do not demand from myself success, approval or the recognition of others.

f) To enjoy nature by returning to it and seeing it, perhaps, for the very first time.

g) To move beyond all of the concepts, conditioning, addictions and attachments I had acquired in life, the drugs, if you like, and learn to be truly free.

Now if somebody had exposed me to this way of thinking when I was much younger, I know I would have responded by saying, '*What a complete load of rubbish'*, but that only serves to prove how conditioned I had been up to that point in my life. So conditioned in fact, that I couldn't even see or recognise what was going on because, and I'll say it again, I had become a *'stranger to myself'*. Ironically, it was easier to cling to that *stranger* than it was to be honest with the one person I knew I needed to be honest with, myself. Yet there came that time in my life when I knew I wanted to be break free and it was all down to me and not someone else. This was something only I could do because it was my life. It's strange to admit it now but the key to everything was becoming *self-aware*, even to my own fears.

'Can you explain that in a different way just to help me understand things a little better please?'

It's like being dead!

'Excuse me?'

Living a life that one day you realise is a lie. That all your life you have allowed yourself to be manipulated, controlled and dominated to the point that you have become someone other than your true self! That you have become so afraid to live that you have become someone else, afraid to be who you really are; is that not like being dead to your true self? That, my friend is what I'm talking about, can you not see that?

'I can now but it sounds so sad!'

It is but it's not the end of the story because once you discover that it is possible to be happy, that you can be your true self and you don't have to be afraid, then that's the day that you start living for the first time. That's the day when the *stranger* you had become starts to die and the real you emerges out into the light.

'MY FEELINGS MATTER!'

CHAPTER FOURTEEN

Sometimes people say they have a *'lightbulb'* moment, when they discover something for the first time. For me, this *'lightbulb'* moment happened when I became *'aware'*. Now and again, and this is purely me talking here, when I describe *'awareness'*, I'm not talking about analysis of any kind but rather *realisation* or more accurately, *self-realisation*. So here is what I call my three step approach:

Step One

Be *aware* of:

- all your illusions about life
- identifying all those things in life you are addicted to but don't really need
- being clear about identifying both your desires and fears
- when you get this, then that's your *'lightbulb'* or 'a*ha*' moment

Step Two

Reflect on:

- giving yourself time – as much time as you need

- continuing to make the effort to understand yourself
- tackling the big questions such as, '*How can I be happy?*' or '*How can I really live?*' or '*How can I be me?*'
- not being afraid to live as **YOU**!

Step Three

Never identify:

- with negative feelings because they are not **YOU**!
- being afraid of getting in touch with your feelings
- but understand and believe that your feelings are real but they are not **YOU**!

This is where I need to explain myself a little bit better when it comes to feelings so hold on and here we go!

My first rule has to be that my feelings are real, they are inside of me and I experience them, so they are real. Never tell me anything different! Right?

'*Right!*'

Now here's the tricky bit so stay with me, okay?

'*Okay.*'

My feelings might be real but they are **NOT ME** or putting it another way, I am not the sum total of my feelings because I am more than that! The minute we identify with our feelings we are on the slippery slope to be being lost.

'How does that work then?'

Here are three examples for you:

'I am lonely.'

'I am disappointed.'

'I am depressed.'

Can you see what I have done here?

'Can't say I can really!'

What I am trying to say is that the mistake I have made is to identify who I am with how I feel. Or putting it another way, I have identified myself with my feelings and as a result, become them. You see feelings come and go. So I might be feeling lonely now but tomorrow, who knows? In the same way, I might be feeling disappointed now but again, tomorrow is another day as they say. In this way, I am accepting my feelings as real because they are and I am experiencing them but I am not allowing them to define, claim and own me. So just like clouds, which come and go, so do my feelings.

I put all of this down to me though and only I can do something about it. This is where true freedom comes in. The freedom which allows me not to be defined by how I feel but who I really am. It was at this point I also became aware of something else. Which was, feeling like this had facilitated within me a propensity to be violent to myself, not in a physical way you understand but in an emotional and psychological sense. The feelings of dissatisfaction, which had built up within me, had led me to a place of damage and brokenness that had become normality for me. After all, didn't everyone feel like this about life or was it just me? At this point, the danger is that you just accept things as they are because there is, literally, no other way to live. Imagine that, becoming lost, giving in to the *stranger I had become'. B*eing a prisoner to my own feelings and never knowing or experiencing what true happiness is. Yet what I am saying here is that it doesn't have to be that way. There is, in fact, another way to live, another way to be and another way to achieve happiness!

You see, ultimately my feelings do matter but I realised that I needed to be able to interpret them, deal with them and see them for what they really are;

part of me but **NOT ME**. When I understood that, I stopped being violent to myself and stepped out of the shadows of the *'stranger'* I had become and started to be the real me.

'ON YOUR MARKS, GET SET, GO!'
CHAPTER FIFTEEN

'Now where did the title for this chapter come from then?'

From my childhood and my earliest memories but I'll explain that in a minute. First, let me emphasise again the importance of *'awareness'* and its vital role in moving forward. For me, awareness means knowing and hopefully understanding what is happening to you. Here I am describing how I became *'aware'* of how I had become a victim to my own past, which was doing me no good whatsoever. Indeed, it was actually causing me harm, damaging me and this is what I meant when I talked about being violent to myself in the last chapter. Equally however, I also recognised within me a desire to experience life in a different way, a way in which I could actually be my true self. However, to achieve this I had to stop being a slave to myself based on my own experiences of the past. The only problem was, as I have said before, continued to be the fact that I knew I was afraid to let go and be myself.

'But where did all of this come from?'

Revisiting your own childhood is never easy at the best of times at least, that is, for me but I knew, somehow, that this was the key to not only getting started but to understanding everything. It seems simple to say this now but I identified the fact that no fear meant no violence and in that way, the endless cycle of unhappiness could be broken. As far back as I can remember, self-dissatisfaction had been ingrained into me. I mentioned in an earlier chapter how:

- competition
- comparisons
- being pushed
- being told you or what you are doing is not good enough

shaped the person I was becoming. So I asked myself, *'Did I really need all that pushing?'* What, in fact, did it ever achieve? The result was inner conflict, a battle if you like, between what I was told to be and who I knew I really was. Let's face it and it's easy to say now, though I couldn't really articulate it at the time, all I wanted to be was happy, to be free to be me, my true self. Nobody ever tells you how to achieve that; nobody ever helps you to be at peace with yourself and to be truly human. Instead, we're fed the diet of competition, comparisons, being told, repeatedly, you're not good enough and being pushed to the point that it really is sink or swim. Is this what life is ultimately all about?

'So what happens?'

From my own point of view, I would say that you end up hating yourself, being discontent with life and this is what I mean by doing violence to yourself. No wonder there are so many people with mental health problems with so much inner conflict being experienced by so many people. It's at this point though, that I learnt a very important lesson and it took me a while to appreciate how vital it was and continues to be and it is this: *Do not fall into the trap of looking for someone or something to blame.* Rather, seek to understand the issues involved, those which have detrimentally affected your well-being, as I have constantly tried to point out in the pages of this book.

'I need a little help with that please.'

Think of it like this. Recognise the inner conflict taking place within you. That is to say, appreciate the battle raging inside of you between who you are told to be and who you know you really are. I call this, as you know, '*awareness*' but equally you could define it in terms of raised consciousness. Equally, the key tool in being able to do this is *sensitivity*, which along with our ability to *empathise* is one of those skills which defines us as human beings. You may have heard of something called '*emotional intelligence*', something which is beyond the scope of this book to explore but today, many people are discovering how understanding this helps them cope with life much better. Indeed, many organisations are identifying highly developed levels of '*emotional intelligence*' as the *key skill* in defining the most important attribute in aspiring leaders. So what I am saying here is this, that eventually I reached the point of being so '*aware*' of my own feelings that I could actually be sensitive to myself. This led me to seeing **FEAR** as the **ONE** thing which prevented me from being my true self and from being truly human. So as a result my mantra became '**Do not be afraid!**'

- Do not be afraid of being who you really are
- Do not be afraid of your own feelings
- Do not be afraid of what you think other people might or might not be thinking of you
- Do not be afraid to do what you want to do or be
- Do not be afraid to take risks

- Do not be afraid to do something new
- Do not be afraid that you might not succeed
- Do not be afraid of life or living

So instead of *'On your marks, get set and go'*, I said to myself, **STOP**!

- Stop making demands on yourself
- Stop having expectations of yourself
- Stop pushing yourself

As I began to understand more and more of the battle raging within myself, I started to learn simply to let go and live. The time had come to nourish myself, to feed on what I needed to survive and to truly live. Then possibly for the first time in my life, I actually began to see everything in a different way. All of a sudden it was perfectly acceptable, no it was fantastic, just to be able to see and enjoy nature. With that I also discovered it was possible to enjoy good company, a book or a movie for their own sake. Finally, I had broken my false addictions and the bars of my prison cell, built entirely by me and referred to previously as the *'captivity of negativity'*, were falling apart. Wow! When that happened I stopped feeding myself on:

- popularity
- appreciation

- praise
- being in control
- having power
- winning the race

I stopped caring what I thought other people were thinking about me; I just stopped! And then I started living! Finally, I could say *'goodbye'* to *'the stranger'* I had become to myself and instead, became who I really am and on that day, I felt, perhaps for the first time in my life, truly alive.

PART TWO

'THE SUN AND THE MOON'

'REBEL - REBEL'
CHAPTER SIXTEEN

From this point on you, the reader, will notice something completely different about this book and my style of writing. This is because I am going to look back over my life and make a number of observations about the times and experiences I have lived through and the impact they have had on my mental health. I cannot say that in every case I was aware of them at the time but on reflection they were to play a significant role in my life. You may not have even heard of some of the people, music, films and television shows I am going to reference in this chapter but each of them in their own and unique way, were to influence how I felt about myself.

So, I am going to start in the early 1970s with someone who was to hugely affect the way I thought about life and the way I viewed myself. The person I am talking about is **David Bowie**. When he emerged onto the scene in the early 1970s, all of a sudden it became clear to me that it was, as a fact, perfectly acceptable just to be you. So you could dress how you liked, have your hair the way you wanted it, behave in a way that was a true reflection of the person you knew yourself to be and ultimately, just be comfortable with yourself! There is a song by David Bowie, which sums this up perfectly and it is called **'Rebel, Rebel!'**. It takes courage to literally break free and to be the person you know yourself deep down to be because, as we have already said, there are so many factors pushing you in the opposite direction. **David Bowie's** whole career was marked by a series of reinventions whereby he pushed back the conventions of society, continually offering different versions of himself to the world. Just as you thought you knew who he was, **Bowie** was brave enough to kill that version off and begin again and again and again. But for me, everything began with the first spectacular invention he came up with about himself, *'Ziggy Stardust'*, summed up in the album, *'The Rise and Fall of Ziggy Stardust and the Spiders from Mars'*.

However, as always, things were not as simple as that. Breaking the mould of convention surrounding you in order to be free does not happen overnight. Indeed, as I found out it can, in fact, be a long, drawn-out and painful process. Growing up in the early

1970s brought with it, as least for me and I suspect for many others the pressure just to conform and be like everybody else. I will not labour a point I have already made in the earlier part of the book but I think we all know that the most difficult person to be in life is, in fact, yourself. Especially when you are continually told '*that's not good enough!*'. There are two songs which sum this scenario up for me, the first being, '*My Perfect Cousin*' by the **Undertones** released in 1980. The cousin in question is Kevin, who comes across as being perfect in every conceivable way, so the message is a simple one and it comes with a question, '*Why can't you just be like your cousin?*'. See what I mean? The second song, '*Why Can't I be You?*', is by the **Cure**, released in 1987 and reflects on the inevitable need to satisfy the longing, that true happiness can only be found by being someone else.

This now brings me back to **David Bowie** who was not afraid to challenge both convention and conformity in how he looked, lived, created and performed. Perhaps the best way to sum this up is in his song '*Changes*' released in 1971. Indeed, so important was this song to him that it was the last one he performed before his retirement in 2006. Change is essential to life, as nothing stands still but as we grow older, we become resistant to change simply because we are afraid of it. But if this happens in the earlier part of our lives then perhaps we will never know, realise, appreciate, recognise or understand our own true potential and how sad is that? **Bowie** challenges such a way of looking at life and paves the way for seeing things differently. It does not mean that you have to wear outrageous clothes and adopt unconventional lifestyles but it is an invitation to, at least, dare to be different or might I even say, '*To dare even to be your true self*'?

When I think back to those days now there was, as I have already alluded to, a tension within me, a battle if you like, going on between the person I felt myself drifting into being and who I knew I really was. The danger with all of this is that you feel trapped and suffocated by life and that is why the song, '*I Want to Break Free*' by **Queen** sums these feelings up perfectly. Of course I wanted to be free to be me, to be the person I knew I was but I was constantly being told '**NO!**'. You had to conform to the expectations of others.

Such tension inevitably gives rise to feelings of both anger and frustration and that is why the **Sex Pistols** with the song, *'Anarchy in the UK'*, released in 1977, resonated so much with the young people of the day. How was it possible to break the mould and in the words of **Queen**, *'break free'*? How was it possible to be yourself, when all the time you were being conditioned to be someone or something else? What kind of mind-set did this create and how was it possible to be healthy in the midst of it?

Personally, I found great solace in two songs of the same name but by different artists. The title of the song in question first of all was, *'Do Anything You Wanna Do'*. The first version was by a band called **Eddy and the Hot Rods,** released in 1977 and was full of vibrant energy. Its message was a simple, if somewhat angry, one that you can do anything you want to do with your own life. You do not have to be told what to do, instead you can choose for yourself because it is your life and no one has the power to manipulate or control you. It takes courage and bravery but stand up for yourself and literally, you can, *'do anything you wanna to do!'*. To be honest I loved that song with its raw, pure and pulsating energy. It had the power to issue an invitation, one that you needed to apply to yourself, which was to take heart, be strong and do it! Two years later in 1979, the band **Thin Lizzy**, one of my all-time favourites if I'm honest, released the single, '***Do Anything You Want To***'. The message was the same but the lyrics resonated powerfully with me as I wrestled with my own sense of identity. Here are some examples:

'There are people that will investigate you,
They'll insinuate, intimidate and complicate you.
People that despise you will analyse then criticise you.
They'll scandalise and tell lies until they realise
You are someone they should have apologised to.
Don't let these people compromise you
Be wise to ...
'You can do anything thing you want to ...'

(Written by Phil Lynott and featured on the album, 'Black Rose: A Rock Legend', released in 1979.)

For me at the time, this was fantastic and liberating stuff but despite this, the struggle went on.

Later in the book I will spend time specifically exploring some of my own pain and suffering but for now, I will do this only in general terms. Yet recognising the prison you are in is one thing, plotting your escape can be something completely different, hence for a while, you just end up experiencing pain and no one knows what you are going through. In many ways, the song '*Running Up That Hill*' by **Kate Bush**, released in 1985, encapsulates this by reflecting on the impossibility of a man being able to actually know and experience how a woman really feels and vice versa. As a result, trapped inside your own pain, struggling to be free, with no one else able to understand or sympathise, does feel like trying to run up an impossibly steep hill. Perhaps that is why looking back and in any way trying to relive those experiences can be extremely painful. For this reason I have always found the song '*Pictures of You*' by **The Cure**, released in 1989, to be extremely powerful. The lyrics reflect on long lost love through the memories conjured up by old photographs and explore the pain, loneliness and isolation experienced as a result. For me you do not need to, literally, physical possess such images because the memories themselves can be enough. The subsequent album by **The Cure**, '*Disintegration*' (1989), provides the listener with a brilliant opportunity for further self-reflection but it is definitely not for the feint hearted.

For now I am going to stay with the pain of not being able to be your true self and reflect a little further on how people may react to you and what consequences this might have for your happiness, well-being and mental health. Back in 1975, I was deeply shocked by a television programme I watched which made a deep impression on me, though at the time I found it difficult to explain why. The programme I am talking about is called, '**The Naked Civil Servant**' and it starred John Hurt as a gay man trying to be, literally, his true self at a time when *most* people struggled with this. I can remember distinctly feeling appalled at the abuse he experienced, both verbal and physical but at the same time, I could not help but respect a man trying to live out, despite all the negativity he experienced, his true identity. In a similar way, the film '**The Elephant Man**', released in 1985 and again staring John Hurt, deeply disturbed me to the point that to this day I struggle to watch it. Filmed entirely in black and white, it explores the life of Joseph Merrick, struck down with a terrible disease which disfigures him. The sadistic, exploitative abuse this fellow human being was subjected to continues to haunt me to this day and is a reminder to us all, not just as a metaphor but also as a real example, as to how low human cruelty to another person can stoop.

You see, when this happens and your life is dominated by fear, one of the options is to escape. As a boy I loved westerns and the song, '***Wild West Hero***' found on the album '***Out of the Blue***' by **ELO** and released in 1977, summed this up perfectly for me. Imagine for one minute being able to escape all of your worries and anxieties. Then imagine being able to go to a place where you mattered, where you could be yourself and find true happiness. This song, therefore, powerfully engendered for me these sentiments and at the same time, defined escapism in its truest sense. As a little boy **J.R.R. Tolkien** conjured up these same feelings for me when I read '**The Hobbit**' for the first time. Imagine being able to go on an adventure, the result of which would mean you would be able to find your true self. The ups and downs of the little and insignificant *Bilbo Baggins* meant that in the end, he not only became the hero but also discovered his true potential. Later I was to find the same truth on a grander scale in '**The Lord of**

the Rings' but the message which came through remained the same, that it was the little and insignificant people who, in the end, would save the day. You see the lesson I was learning from all of this was to be strong, be brave, take courage and never lose heart but at the same time - *just be yourself.* Yes there will be pain, suffering and hardship but it will not last forever and in the end, all will be well.

This brings me to the song by **Bob Marley**, *'Three Little Birds'* released in 1977 with the lyrics, *'Don't worry about a thing, because everything little thing, is gonna to be all right'*. Easy to say 'I know' but sometimes we need that light in the darkness, we need hope, we need to believe that the bad times cannot continue forever and this song sums up these sentiments to perfection. You see, there comes that moment when you are ready to break free, to break the chains of your own self-imposed prison cell, to walk out of the shadows and leave the *'stranger to yourself'* you had become behind; for good. When you make that decision, you cannot look back and you cannot afford to have any regrets because it is a question, literally, of now or never. So my final song is by **Queen** and it is called, *'**Don't Stop Me Now**'* (1979) and I can't think of a better way to end this chapter than with these most appropriate of words.

Chapter Play List

- 'Rebel - Rebel' – David Bowie
- 'My Perfect Cousin' – The Undertones
- 'Why Can't I Be You?' – The Cure
- 'Changes' – David Bowie
- 'I Want To Break Free' – Queen
- 'Anarchy In The UK' – The Sex Pistols
- 'Do Anything You Wanna Do' – Eddy and the Hot Rods
- 'Do Anything You Want To' – Thin Lizzy
- 'Running Up That Hill' – Kate Bush
- 'Pictures of You' – The Cure
- 'Wild West Hero' – The Electric Light Orchestra
- 'Three Little Birds' – Bob Marley
- 'Don't Stop Me Now' – Queen

'DON'T LOOK BACK IN ANGER'

CHAPTER SEVENTEEN

'Slip inside the eye of your mind,
Don't you know you might find
A better place to play ...' (Oasis)

This is going to be the hardest chapter for me to write so far. The reason for this is that it will involve pain - personal pain. You see, I need to share with you some of my experiences of life so that you will know how I have been shaped and formed by what I, personally, have gone through. To do this, I need to go back and revisit much of my childhood where most of the pain can be found. All I can say at this stage is that it had a profound effect on me and consequently, proved to dominate much of the person I have become.

My style will be a simple one in so far as I will adopt an episodic narrative by recalling a series of childhood memories that I will share with you. I will explain the title of the chapter towards the end but for now, I will let the experiences speak for themselves. As I said, it will not be easy. In fact, I know that it will be extremely painful but for me, it is something I need to do if I am to explain fully where many of my thoughts and feelings about life have come from. Here we go then ...

She

She came from a family of seven, with two sisters and four brothers, living on a small farm in County Mayo in the West of Ireland. The house was one of those whitewashed, almost picture-postcard type cottages, that you often see on biscuit tins and the like. Life, however, was far from romantic living in such a harsh environment. There was no electricity and no gas with the sole source of cooking and heating being the peat-fuelled fire, which was the centre of the home. There was one main living space, which contained a table and a small alcove separated from the rest of the room by a curtain. This served as her parent's bedroom, providing some degree of privacy. The children, on the other hand, often slept in a single room with the boys and the girls in two separate beds. Life on the farm was harsh with early morning starts, long walks to school and all the necessary chores that needed to be completed if they were ever going to survive, especially the long cold winters. At school, she learned to read, write and do basic mathematics but that was about it. The driving force was to earn your keep as soon as possible. The only problem being that there were no jobs, outside the farm, for miles around. Eventually it became impossible for the family to exist and support nine individuals, so with no employment in the local area, one by one her sisters and brothers looked across the water to England for a better life.

Eventually, this was where she gazed too and with high expectations of a new and better life, she set off for the industrial city of Birmingham where employment was more or less guaranteed. How different life must have looked in this new cosmopolitan city with its dance halls, cinemas and well-dressed locals. With the little money she had managed to save, she found a small room to rent and work in a nearby factory. Now, perhaps for the first time in her life, she could actually live in a comfortable way. Yet she never forgot where she came from and always sent money back to the 'old country' for her parents to help them stave off the harsh realities of life on the farm. So, with money in her pocket and a smile on her face, she could at last afford to buy herself the odd treat, perhaps a handbag or a pair of earrings, a new skirt or a cardigan and even a night out on the town. For the most part, she stuck with those she knew which meant the other Irish immigrants who flooded the inner parts of Birmingham making the slum areas their own. After all, who else would want to live there? Huge crowds would gather after Mass on a Sunday to catch up on life back at home and to feel part of something bigger than themselves. She was making a new life for herself and it must have felt good.

Then one day, she met somebody and they fell in love. He received instructions in the Catholic faith and they were married soon after. They say that love is blind but I cannot help but wonder: did she really know what she was letting herself in for? The man she married was a veteran of the Second World War and in ways few of us can ever begin to imagine, was broken by his experiences there. I have no doubt that, at first, they were happy and not long after they were married they had their first child, a son, followed by a daughter then sadly a miscarriage. You see her husband was a heavy drinker possibly his way of coping and breaking down the memories that followed him home from the war. But alcohol brings with it much more than just the drink. There were those times when, in the morning, after a heaving drinking session the night before, he simply could not get up to go to work the next day. Who would put food on the table and clothes on the children's' backs then? Then came the gambling! Again, was it to forget? Was it for the thrill? Or was it just a distraction from what life had become? Perhaps it was all these things but whatever the truth was, things began to spiral out of control. There were arguments, fights, late nights, debt, times when he would not come home at all or even not be seen for days. What was she to do now?

The most precious thing in life to her was her children and she would do whatever it took to provide for them. So now, she was forced to do what she had always done, work. Sometimes it was cleaning, sometimes it was in a factory, sometimes it was both but day in and day out, she would work and work and work, almost to the point of physical and mental exhaustion. Her sole motivation was to provide for her two children. She would be the one to make sure that they had the right school uniform. She would be the one to make sure that they were fed and nourished. She would be the one to make sure that life for them would be as normal as it could be when in reality, it was far from that. Gone now were the earrings, handbags and *the odd treat. Instead, the only luxury she allowed herself was cigarettes and these were eventually to lead to her death.*

Life for her then was not easy. It never had been and it never would be again, that was just the way it was. The children struggled. The boy became pasty looking and seriously underweight, to the point that the doctors had to send him for sunray treatment. There he would sit, bare-chested, with goggles on in front of a sunray lamp along with several other boys, in an attempt to reverse a serious deficiency in vitamin D. They found it hard to make progress at school because of the late nights they had to endure along with the arguments, fights and disagreements over money. Sometimes, the rent failed to be paid or they fell into arrears over something they had been forced to buy on credit. There were no holidays, no central heating, no telephone, no car, no luxuries; just existence if you could call it that. And all the while she continued to work.

Certain things in life you can only put up with for so long until in the end, they grind you down. Day-by- day, month-by-month, year-by-year, hoping that things would improve, maybe get better even but they rarely do. In the end, life just beats you. You run out of energy.

It happens slowly but you start to get weak. In the past, you fell down but you knew, she knew, you had to get up again. There was no other option but one day, you fall and you just cannot get back up. Do not get me wrong, you want to but your strength has gone, it has been consumed by life. Now the weight is just too heavy to bear anymore. You see, her children had grown up, now they were standing on their own two feet, her job was complete and it was time to let go. At first it was a stroke, which confined her to bed, then the weakness and the cruelty of life just simply overwhelmed her. Her son took the hand she could no longer use and rubbed it gently down the side of his face. She smiled and one tear left the corner of her eye and rolled gently down her cheek. The lines on her face told her story but only he could read it. It was time to let go now. Her strength was gone and she had nothing more to give. She closed her eyes for the last time and would never open them again in this life. Now it was the turn of her son to wipe the tears away from his face but he knew her story and one day, when the time was right, he would tell it.

If you have not worked it out already I have just told you the story of my own mother and what I need to do now, is go back into that life and relive some of the memories I have with you. The approach I will take is a simple one with no particular chronology. Instead, I will offer a series of, what might best be described as, '*flash-backs*' each of which will describe a traumatic event from my childhood. The one word, however, which will bind them all together is 'pain'.

PAIN
'Slippers on the wrong feet!'

It was a rare occurrence but my mother had actually gone out for the evening, leaving my sister and me in the house with our father alone. I remember the coal fire burning in the hearth, its warm glow throwing out comforting heat into the darkened room. The furniture sparse but comfortable, the night cold but dry. I was wearing thin, baggy pyjamas, perhaps a size or two too large for me, my dressing gown thrown over a nearby chair. I recall feeling very sleepy and my father picking me up, pushing two armchairs together and placing me gently down between them. I was asleep in seconds. Then I woke up, my eyes shot open and I knew there was something wrong and I didn't quite know what. Pushing the chairs aside, I looked around the room expecting to see my dad but found nothing. Now here's the thing, I distinctly remember putting my slippers on but on the wrong feet! I remember putting my dressing gown on and wrapping the chord around my waist and I remember panicking. After all, where was my dad?

Imagine that, waking up at about three or four years of age only to find you were in the house by yourself. I do not recall, however, having any memories about my sister or her whereabouts at all at this point. The only feelings I remember having, in fact, were ones of fear, complete loneliness and panic. Convincing myself that the house was empty, I ran out of the front door and down the garden path in what felt like to me, at least, was the middle of the night. My slippers remained, somehow, firmly on the wrong feet but by now I was really frightened and the only thing I knew I had to do was find my dad. I came to a main road. I don't know how I got across, I just did because all I knew was that on the other side of that road, there were lights on and that meant the '*pub*' and, hopefully, my dad. To this day, the name of that '*pub*' is burned into my memory: '*The Lodge*'. I pushed at the heavy doors but they barely moved until someone opened them from the inside. Looking up, I stared into the eyes of what looked like a very fierce man, his face full of creases and lines and his breath fresh with the smell of stale alcohol. "What do want?" he asked.

'My dad,' I replied. By now, my chin had begun to wobble and my little eyes were full of tears. I am a little unclear as to what exactly happened next but I do recall how the '*pub*' itself was full of sound, largely the deep and heavy voices of men, the air full of cigarette smoke and the smell, that of stale beer. Somebody must have recognised me because my dad emerged out of the crowd, picked me up and carried me home.

That memory has stayed with me all these years. Sometimes when I ask myself, 'What is the source of all your vulnerability and where did it come from?', my mind takes me back to that night and the little boy who, in the darkness, woke up only to discover that he was in the house all by himself and that he put his slippers on the wrong feet in order to go and find his dad.

'Fire, Fire!'

This is hard to imagine but once again, it is one of those experiences burned so deep into my memory that even to think of it now makes me want to stop writing. One night, my dad came home extremely drunk and angry. He'd had an argument with a publican and been thrown out. Effectively he had been barred which, to be honest, was not uncommon. Anyway, staggering home he came in, demanding money from my mum and looking for a bottle and some rags. His intention was to go back out, buy some petrol and bomb the '*pub*'. Mum pleaded with him not to go but his mind was made up and he wouldn't listen. So armed with cash, several bottles and some rags, he set off in search of the nearest petrol station. *What were we supposed to do now?* We did not know the name of the '*pub*' so that was not an option. Instead, my mum made my sister and I put our coats on top of our pyjamas and we set off in search of the nearest petrol station. I do not know what time it was but it must have been very late, as the streets were all dark and empty.

We tramped from one petrol station to the next, warning them not to sell any petrol to a man wanting it in a bottle. My mum was worried out of her wits as my sister and I held on to her hands, one on each side, walking the streets, not really knowing what to expect, not really knowing what to do or where to turn. In the end we made our way home, Mum making my sister and I go to bed while she stayed up waiting for Dad to come home. Eventually he returned, at what hour I do not know. He never mentioned the incident again but the stress and anxiety it caused remains with me to this day.

As I mentioned earlier in the chapter, we lived in a small, back-to-back house, which the local authority eventually decided to condemn as unfit for human habitation and then demolish. It would be a systematic removal of poor housing whilst at the same time, moving the deserving residents to better accommodation within the city. As a result, many of the houses around ours were flattened but we still remained. At one point behind where we lived, the whole area had been cleared and some youths had decided it would be a good idea to gather together all of the available rotting wood, place it against the wall and set fire to it. The only problem with this was that the wall they had chosen backed on to where we lived.

Once again, I distinctly remember Dad coming home drunk and thankfully going to bed early. Then in the middle of the night, Mum woke us up because there was obviously a problem. I remember feeling hot and smelling the smoke but it seemed so far away. At this point, Mum tried to raise Dad but he was too far-gone and he literally would not move. We all stood there in the bedroom trying to rouse him, doing all we could from pulling him, removing the bed clothes and shouting, to crying and screaming, all to no avail. Can you imagine what it must have been like standing in a room, separated by the flames of a roaring fire only by a brick wall, with tendrils of thick, black smoke invading the air, believing that your dad was, literally, going to die and that you could do nothing about it! To scream, *'Fire, Fire!'* at the top of your voice, eyes full of tears and to be met only with silence, would be a traumatic experience for anyone, let alone a mother and her two very young children. Those moments felt like an eternity to that little boy but in the end, the fire service arrived and my dad, oblivious to everything, slept right through it all.

'Christmas Time – Mistletoe and Wine'

You may recognise the title of this reflection from the Christmas song by the well-known and much-loved Sir Cliff Richard. I have chosen it because I have a love/hate relationship with this, '*Most Wonderful Time of the Year*'. I love Christmas for all the reasons most people do, so let me share with you now some of the reasons why I still struggle to enjoy the '*festive season,*' when everyone is supposed to be full of joy and hope.

It was Christmas Eve and my mother, my sister and I were waiting up for Dad to return home from the '*pub*'. It was very late when through a crack in the curtain, we saw him staggering from one side of the road to the other as he made his way home. By the time he reached the front door, he did not have the co-ordination skills to put the key in the lock and so Mum had to open it for him. I remember feeling very nervous, as none of us quite knew what to expect but to be honest, that was fairly normal for us. Sometimes he would go straight to bed but when he sat down in his armchair and looked straight at us, I knew then that things were going to literally '*kick off*'. I cannot use the foul and abusive language that came out of his mouth here, nor can I adequately describe how terrified we all were. All I can say is that he was hell-bent on starting, and by that I mean arguing. I had learnt that over the years, the best thing to do was to never to get into an argument with him because that only made things worse. Tonight, however, he was adopting a different approach. "After what I've seen tonight," he said, "I might never go out again!"

What exactly he had seen, he never said but in different ways, he kept on repeating the same thing over and over again. None of us, of course, believed anything that he said as we all knew that in the morning he would have forgotten everything. Then all of a sudden, he jumped up and made for the sideboard. Opening the drawer, he found what he was looking for: a small bottle of holy water and proceeded to walk around the room, sprinkling us with it. By now it was well past midnight, on Christmas Eve, a night when all children are supposed to be tucked up in bed, struggling to get to sleep in anticipation of the great day to come. Yet here we were, sitting in a cold room in the early hours of the morning, being sprinkled with holy water by a man using foul and abusive language. Perhaps now you can begin to understand why, to this day, I still struggle to enjoy Christmas. That year though, I was to experience one of the moments which I referred to earlier in this book as *'awareness'*. It happened when I picked up a small, plastic figure of Father Christmas. I cannot remember where it came from now but I swore to myself that I would keep it, to remind me of that night and in the future, to do everything I could to make sure that such things would never happen again. One of the things about Christmas I used to enjoy the most was that the *'pubs'* were closed and if Dad stayed in and was sober, we could have at least a taste of what a normal Christmas was like. However, there were times when he always knew which *'pubs'* did, in fact, open their doors even on Christmas Day. I can recall him going out relatively late and coming home early but I have no recollections of him behaving badly on the big day itself. It is just that for one day in the year, it would have been really nice to enjoy a trouble-free, family, Christmas.

If you can recall the first part of this chapter when I focused on my mother, we were always relatively poor. Our furniture tended to be cheap and well-used. There were no carpets on the floor and often the rugs that we had were threadbare. I can recall one bitterly cold winter in the season of Christmas, coming down stairs and finding Dad sitting in his armchair by the fire in his underwear. He had been out drinking the night before and was still under the influence of alcohol and for that reason he never saw me, but what he did deeply saddened me. Sitting there with his head bowed forward, I watched him spit onto the threadbare rug before proceeding to rub it in with his foot. I remember thinking that we had nothing of value and no prospect of things improving, so why do this to the little that we had? It made no sense then and it makes no sense now. To this day, I have to try really hard if I am to rise to the challenge that Christmas still presents. Such memories continue to haunt me and there is still much to come.

'Shout, Shout – let it all out!'

There have been times, I must confess, both then and now that I have literally wanted to rage against the injustice and unfairness of it all. It was not the poverty, as far as I was concerned, back in the day. At least, not where I lived, because as far as I knew everyone was in the same boat. No, it was more than that, it was the sense not only that you were being kicked when you were down but you were being stomped on afterwards too. What follows now is a series of short reflections, each of which encapsulates my need to '**Shout, Shout and let it all out**'. Hopefully you will see what I mean.

Friday was payday for my dad and we always went shopping to the local supermarket as a family. Of course, we walked everywhere and it was a fair distance to where we needed to go. One such venture has stuck in my mind because from the moment we stepped out of the house to the moment we came back, Mum and Dad never stopped arguing. I cannot remember the details. All I can recall is the foul and abusive language that went to and fro between them. Can you imagine for one second how that made two small children feel, as they gripped their parent's hands, marching along a busy street in full view of everyone? I remember thinking then, '*Why did it have to be this way and why didn't anyone seem to care?*' When the arguing stopped I cannot recall but as always, nobody came to help.

My sister and I had a strong, black money box supplied, I think, by the local bank. What I do know, however, is that the only way it could be opened was for the box, hopefully full of coins, to be taken to the bank where a special key would be used to release the accumulated treasure. For the most part, this would have been pennies but an occasional sixpence, a 'thrupenny bit' or even a shilling, would be placed through the small slit in the side of the box. You can imagine how excited I was at the thought of one day making that journey to the bank and to be given some money that was actually my own, so that I could buy anything I wanted! However, one day Dad came home looking for money, either for drink, gambling or both. Finding my mum's purse empty, he made for the moneybox, took it down into the cellar and smashed it with a hammer, until literally all of the coins tumbled out. Gathering them up, he left the house without looking back. If he had turned his head, even for a second, he would have seen a little boy, tears streaming down his face, staring at a smashed money box, knowing that in that moment the few dreams he had for the future had now been broken too.

Years later, another incident happened involving money. By now I was receiving a small amount of pocket money, which as young people do, I tended to spend as soon as possible. However, it did generate a certain amount of change, small coins, that I kept in a drawer in my bedroom. One morning when I was still in bed, Dad came quietly into my room, opened the drawer and took anything of value. He never said anything about the incident and neither did I but once again, I was left with those feelings of desperately wanting to know why.

Staying on the theme of my bedroom, another incident which I can clearly recall, still fills my heart with much sadness and sorrow. This time it was in the middle of the night and I woke up as my dad entered the room. Clearly he had lost his way and was disorientated but what happened next broke my heart in two. At first I was not sure what was going on, as there appeared to be a silent pause before I heard what sounded like running water. Half asleep and confused, it suddenly hit me as to what was actually going on. Dad was, in fact, urinating all over my stuff in the corner of the room. Once again I was too frightened to either say or do anything, so I hid beneath the bed sheets and uttered a silent scream to a world, I knew, was not listening and did not care.

Broken

I must say I am finding it increasingly difficult to share such powerful and emotional experiences with others. Many of the experiences I have described so far, I have never shared with anyone else before; even members of my own family. However, I feel I must do so in the hope that somehow they might be of help to someone else and it is this, which is my primary motivation to keep writing. I am now going to describe a series of incidents which I have called '*Broken*', because that is the best word I can think of to describe the impact they had on me. All these experiences and the trauma they brought with them had a profound effect on my own sense of identity and hopefully by now, you can begin to see the connection between them and what I wrote about being a '*stranger to myself*' in the earlier part of the book. In many ways, I can almost hear myself saying, '*Be someone else. This life you are living is too hard, too unbearable.*'

As a little boy I had a group of teddy bears that I played regularly with. I had collected them over the years. Many of them, like me, were broken with missing eyes, floppy arms or with the stuffing coming out but I saw them, in one sense, as my friends. I gave them names, lined them to watch me play and from time to time would play-fight with them. It was all innocent, good, clean, fun, the kind of thing children do all over the world. Then one afternoon, Dad came home drunk and saw me playing with my teddy bears. For some reason that started him off: *'What was I doing at my age playing with teddy bears? Was I a 'puff' was something wrong with me, was I stupid? I should grow up and throw those bears away!'*. Can you imagine how that made me feel? Can you imagine what it is like when your own dad ridicules you, embarrasses you and shames you? Can you imagine what effect that might have on how you might think about yourself?

One night when I was very young I suddenly woke up because I heard the sound of a loud slap in the darkness. It was the only time I can remember Dad raising a hand directly to my mum. So I ran as fast as I could to her to offer what protection was possible but was told to *'Get out!'*. I ran to where my sister was still asleep and hid alone, in the dark, inside her wardrobe. Surrounded by the darkness, I closed my eyes tightly shut, curled up into a little ball and hoped that I could simply shut out the world.

As you can imagine, Dad would often stay out very late and as a result, my mum would send my sister and I to bed, especially if we had school the next day. Naturally we did not want to go, as our presence would sometimes act as a deterrent to him behaving badly. Sleep, when it did come, would not do so easily and to this day, I still have the habit of waking up at the slightest noise. For this reason I struggle to be able to tolerate mumbled voices at a distance, especially when I am I bed. This is because when Dad did come home I always woke up, staying awake for hours, listening to their voices through the wall, making out the odd word and waiting for the moment when I knew I would have to jump out of bed and rush to the rescue. Needless to say it rarely happened because I was simply too afraid. There are things, however, I heard through that wall, things which even to this day I do not have the emotional strength to put down on paper. This is how I know that part of me is still broken.

Staying quiet though was a skill my mum, sister and I all developed as a way of preserving some quality of life. On those rare occasions when Dad came in, had his dinner and went to bed, we knew that staying quiet was the key to not waking him up. If we could do that then there was a chance he would not go out again and we might all be able to go to bed in peace for once. This meant, however, that the television or radio volume had be turned right down or not used at all. Play was reduced to that which required the minimum of noise and we had to hope against all hope that no one would come to the door. One particular incident stands out for me though and it goes like this:

The night is cold and I find myself in a double bed with my sleeping father. He has come home drunk again and after a series of arguments, we have all been made to go to bed. Essentially, although we have two bedrooms, one is an attic and no one can sleep in there because it is too damp and wet. My sister, my mother and I are all frightened in case the tiniest movement or slightest sound might wake him up and the arguments start all over again. I cannot sleep because I am literally too scared. I cannot help running over in my mind, time and time again, 'What if he wakes up? What if he starts shouting again? What if he hurts us?' Then there is movement in the darkness. I flinch because I cannot see anything. It is too dark and I know someone is there, but who is it? Then a warm hand takes mine and I know who it is – Mum. There, kneeling by the side of the bed, in the darkness, in the cold, wearing a thin nightdress but holding my hand is Mum. That reassurance, with no words being necessary, told me that everything would be all right.'

What kind of life, though, was this and what effect was it having, long term, on my mum, my sister and me?

'I'm Hungry!'

As I said earlier, it felt like we were all poor back in those days but certain things made our situation worse. Dad often went from one job to another. If he had been out the night before, then it was not unusual for him to be unable to get up and go to work the next day As a result, he would more often than not lose his job. Even when he had employment, if he did not feel like going he would simply set off in the morning as usual, leave his overalls on the back of the door of the outside toilet and spend the rest of day either in the '*pub*' or in the betting shop. Mum, of course, was devastated when she found his overalls because no job meant, quite simply, no money and no money meant no food to put on the table. As a result, I can often remember being fed a dish of hot milk containing bread with a layer of white sugar on the top.

On another occasion, the cupboard was literally bare. We had nothing left at all to eat and Mum's purse, at the same time, was completely empty. So there we were on a Friday evening sitting on a wall, our stomachs rumbling with hunger, waiting for Dad to emerge from the factory in which he worked with his wage packet. Thankfully on that occasion he came out and we made our way to the local fish and chip shop for an emergency supper.

However, there were those occasions when Dad had not been to work and so there was no job, which meant no money, which meant no food. As a result, I recall even now, more than once, being taken to the local pawnbrokers. Sometimes it would be his watch, on other occasions a ring he might have but the one standout visit for me was when Dad pawned his war medals. I had little comprehension of what was going on at the time but I remember that event distinctly. It was an emergency trip to get money for food but guess where we went to first on the way home? The *'pub'*!

Many years later, when my sister got married, I had a quiet word with Dad beforehand whereby I asked, or rather pleaded with him not to drink to excess. He told me that he had no money, so I was not to worry and like a fool, I took some consolation in that. His problem as with all alcoholics,, is that once you have had one drink you cannot stop. I did my best to keep an eye on him but inevitably at the reception we were separated. When, eventually, I did catch up with him he opened his wallet, removed a five-pound note and waved it at me, at which point my heart sank.

I will offer one more reflection here, staying on theme of food and drink. I have already mentioned that in the small, back-to-back house in which we lived there was an attic. However, there was a hole in the roof through which you could see the sky! As a result, my father placed a metal bath beneath it to catch the rainwater. One summer he had the idea that perhaps this could become a bedroom for my sister and myself. The only problem was we both hated it and would cry not to be put in there, especially with the door closed. His solution was to feed us with whiskey on a teaspoon in the hope that the alcohol would eventually send us to sleep and at which point he could go out and so it goes on!

Fear

I am entering a phase in this book now, the contents of which I have never shared with anyone else in my life before. It is taking all my emotional strength to do so but I feel I must if I am to give a true picture of not only what formed me, but of the person I eventually became. The one word which dominates, is that of **FEAR** because I was, literally, afraid of everything.

From a very early age I suffered from two things, which I know now are both manifestations of trauma. The first was sleepwalking. Very often I would just get up in the middle of the night, put my dressing gown and slippers on and go for a walk. I would open doors, walk down stairs, go outside and even pick things up, all without any conscious awareness, at all, of what I was doing. Perhaps I was trying to escape, run away even; perhaps my unconscious mind was trying to find a better life somewhere else. Eventually, after many years it just stopped but I often think back to those days and ask myself what did it all really mean?

The second trauma I need to share was my habit of bed-wetting. Once again this goes right back to my earliest memories of waking up morning after morning on wet sheets in wet pyjamas. At the time, it was extremely embarrassing and I wanted no one else to know because this was something I needed to keep private and I was desperate to do so. Every time I wet the bed I was asleep, so it was not something I was conscious of and therefore, I was not doing it deliberately. Sadly, Dad did not see it that way and he would often tell me off for being dirty! Then one day something happened and I will never ever forget it. I suddenly woke up as I was actually wetting the bed and I just lay there; I did not get up, I did not stop, I did not call out. Instead, I just lay there until my bladder was completely empty. However, I did realise something, which was that I was too afraid to get out of bed, too afraid of making a noise, too afraid of waking Dad up, too afraid of breaking the peace and too afraid of all the possible consequences of putting one foot on the floor. It was easier if I just stayed where I was, a broken and afraid little boy lying in his own urine.

Eventually and after many years, I did stop wetting the bed but that was far from the end of the trauma and I now need to explain why. Whilst I was still very young, my life became totally dominated by fear. I had my own small bedroom, which from time to time I had to share with my dad. Mum often used to send my sister and I to bed relatively early when we had to go to school the next day, even though Dad had not returned home from the *'pub'* yet. I remember always trying my hardest to stay awake until he returned home, just in case Mum needed me; it was then that I heard those mumbled voices through the wall. As I said earlier, there were things I heard which are still too painful for me to think about let alone record on paper, even today all these years later. Be that as it may, I had another problem and that was going to the toilet. I was literally too terrified to leave my bedroom so I developed a habit, one that I have never told anyone about in my life before. In my bedroom there was a small rug. I would go to a corner of that rug and urinate; very often it would only take the form of a small trickle. However, I was conscious of the smell so the next time I would go to another corner and do the same, repeating the practice as often as I needed to until all was quiet. Most of the time, I did not need to go to the toilet at all but I convinced myself I did and so the habit continued night after night. It was, of course, a reflection of the nervous state I was in and reveals how much I was both broken and afraid. I often think of that little boy in the darkness of the night, his life dominated by fear, hearing mumbled voices through the wall, convincing himself that he needed to go to the toilet again and again and again.

Now I will come to my final experience, which will once again, further illustrate how my life was dominated by fear. You see, school for me was to become a major problem and here I am talking about junior school, so I am guessing I would have been about seven years old. I can remember thinking even now, all these years later, what might happen to Mum if I went to school and who would be there to protect her. So I cried and I begged not to be sent to school but, of course, there was no choice; I had to go. I remember sitting at a desk all by myself, literally sobbing my heart out, unable to explain to anyone why I felt like that. Part of me was ashamed and of course, part of me just could not put into words what I was feeling. To me the pain was real and the fear crippling. Little was I to know, however, that the teacher I met that day was to change my life forever but I will leave explaining that until later. For now, there was no way out and I was trapped in my own pain, misery, isolation and absolute fear.

I said right at the beginning of this chapter that I would explain the meaning of the title later, so here it is. The song, '***Don't look back in anger***' by **Oasis,** sums up perfectly for me the advice I gave to myself a long time ago. You see, and this might sound strange, I have no doubt that my dad loved me and that he also loved my mum and my sister. Life for him had been hard but he rarely spoke about it. One night, for example, his own father kicked to death a puppy right before the eyes of my dad and his younger brother. Can you imagine witnessing that and what effect it might have on you? In another incident, his father smashed a man over the back of the head with a hammer in a local '*pub*'. Violence, therefore, was a natural part of his life and this was to continue when he joined the army at just sixteen years of age during the Second World War. The sights that he saw formed images in his mind that would never go away. Seeing your best friend having his head blown off, watching as members of your unit are decimated by enemy machine gun fire and being wounded twice, must have profoundly affected him in all kinds of different ways. These were the things I was to learn later in life but they never excused what he put my sister, my mother and myself through. However, I knew that I could not '**look back in anger**' because of what that would have done to me. My own experiences have never gone away and at times, they still haunt me but **anger** is not a word I would use to describe them. Yet sometimes I feel compelled to ask, '*Why, Dad, did you dress up so smartly and spend so much time getting ready just to go out to the pub, leaving your family behind in that poor and run-down house? Why, Dad, did you laugh and joke with your friends, only to come home and abuse your family who had done nothing wrong? Why could you not see the pain and misery you were causing to those closet to you? Why did you never, ever refer to all those times you ranted and raged at us when you eventually came home? What did any of us ever do to deserve treatment like that?*' You see, I cannot dwell on questions such as these for too long because the danger is they conjure up too much pain and too much heartache, even now.

I could not tell you how many public houses, over the years, I have spent outside, usually with my sister and mother. However, I do remember, even when I was very young, making a conscious decision not to go inside them if I was given the choice. Equally, I also made the decision never to drink alcohol or gamble because of the devastating effect they both had upon me. I could continue in this chapter to further recall events from my childhood, like when my Dad smashed open the gas and electric meter boxes to get his hands on the coins inside. The police came to the house and my mother persuaded my dad to admit the crime, which eventually went to court. He *'got off'* however, because he managed to convince the judge that he needed the money to buy food and clothing for his children!

As I come to the end of, what has been for me, a most exhausting but absolutely necessary chapter, I need to reflect on the consequences of my experiences for the person I became. I have called this book '**A Stranger to Myself**' and I often think, '*When did this happen?*' At what stage in my life did I lose who I really am? The answer to this is, of course, extremely complex but in many ways reflecting back now on such dark, lonely and isolating experiences, part of me needs to recognise that I never really lost my true self, it just felt like I did. The only problem with this, as I have stated repeatedly in the first part of the book, is finding your way back.

So, I would have to say that such experiences, over time, shaped me into someone I did not want to be but there was no way to fight it. A frail, vulnerable and frightened little boy was at the mercy of the waves that threatened to engulf him; only later would he learn how to surf. For now though, I could see myself becoming socially distant, not trusting people, fearing confrontation and lacking any kind of self-confidence or belief. As a result, I had a very low sense of self-worth and self-esteem. My life was one dominated and controlled by fear and there was, literally, nothing I could do about it. The only thing I do know is that I would have given anything for my dad, whether in word or deed but preferably both, to have picked me up, hugged me and told me that he loved me. If I could go back now and find that little boy hiding behind a chair in the living room, something he always did whenever visitors came, simply because he was afraid. I would pick him up myself, hold him in my arms and tell him I would never let him go.

'DON'T GIVE UP!'

CHAPTER EIGHTEEN

The name of this final chapter comes from a song by *Peter Gabriel* and features *Kate Bush*. It sums up perfectly what I now want to say and how to leave you, the reader, as I come to the end of my journey. So is there a happy ending then, I ask myself? I think we all know that life, in fact, is not like that. The events I have described in the pages of this book and the experiences I have shared do not end with the words *'and he lived happily ever after'* However, what I have to say now is not all doom and gloom but rather windows into hope.

Over the years I have picked up fragments of my life, a bit like pieces from a jigsaw puzzle, which by themselves do not make sense but when I begin to put them together, a recognisable pattern begins slowly to emerge. Let me give you an example. For as long as I can remember, I have always sympathised with anyone who is left out, pushed to the margins, those who are rejected, despised, unwanted or unloved. As a result, I have felt compelled to do whatever I can to get alongside them, offering help, encouragement and support. I have always put this down to a sort of natural instinct but now I know better. You see, in them I saw myself, the little boy always on the outside looking in and the one to whom no help came because it felt simply like no one cared. In this way, I was able to identify a desperate need within myself to compensate for my own sense of isolation and alienation. Putting it simply, if no one else would help then I would. Such an approach has become so engrained within me that it has become a natural part of who I am. Yet would I have been such a person if I had, in fact, lived a different life with different experiences? Today I find myself embracing this aspect of my personality as the real me and not, therefore, some distant *stranger*. In many ways, I would say it has made me more human but equally it has emerged out of much pain, misery and suffering. With this in mind, I now want to share with you a few rays of sunshine without which my life may well have taken a completely different course.

'Suffer the children'

Let me take you back now to that little boy sitting at his desk in school, sobbing his heart out at the thought that something terrible might happen to his mum while he was away from her. In this book, I deliberately have not included any specific names and I will continue with that approach now, although part of me desperately wants to do so. You see on that day, little was I to know that in that room would be one of the teachers who would change my life forever. Her kind and gentle approach touched my heart in ways that I cannot put into words but almost without me having to say anything, I knew she understood. I was behind in everything but mainly reading and this was something she would put right. Maybe she saw something in me, recognising something I did not know even existed but it was there, lying dormant for someone else to wake up. The first thing she did was to make me feel safe and secure, that school was a place where you could actually relax and be yourself. So all I did first of all was play. As a result, school became a place where I actually wanted to go and dare I say, enjoy. I started to make friends, pick up books and almost without knowing it, began to learn.

The first thing this remarkable woman identified that I needed help with was my reading, so she arranged that I left the class and along with a group of other children, I had extra lessons. Here the teacher spent time with you, identifying your specific needs and nurturing you with calmness and what I can only describe as love. Suddenly, I loved reading and made huge progress over a relatively short period of time. There was a cupboard in the room that contained a selection of books, which the teacher only let you access when you had reached a certain stage in your reading. It became my ambition, one day, to have one of those books because for me, unbelievably, you were also allowed to take them home. Eventually I achieved what had seemed impossible and I was actually allowed to open the cupboard door myself and choose any book I wanted. What a day that was and I will never forget it because it would be a transformational moment in my life. Yet I owe everything to that teacher who took that small, terrified and sobbing little boy into her arms and loved him. It engendered feelings of not being alone anymore and perhaps, most importantly of all, it showed me that there were people who cared in this world after all.

As time went by, school for me at least, became a place of safety and security, almost like a refuge where for a while I could leave the horrors of my life at home behind. I continued to make friends, learned how to play and love football but perhaps most importantly of all, my love for reading thrived. At home there were no books and I can never remember my parents reading, though I do have memories of my mother listening to me read. However, do not get me wrong, my home life did not improve, in fact it was as bad as ever. For that reason, I could never invite friends back to the house to play because the risk of my dad being drunk and causing an embarrassing scene was too great. As a result, a tremendous pressure built up inside of me to keep that part of my life as secret as possible. Little did I know that such an approach to life would later have devastating consequences for my well-being. For now though, I was perfectly happy to walk the tightrope of keeping my life at school and my life at home as separate as possible.

Moving on a few years, something remarkable happened again at school, without any kind of warning at all. The teachers, by now, must have seen something in me worth pushing because they made a decision to move me up a year so that I would spend two years instead of one in my final year at junior school. The reason for this was to have longer to prepare for an examination called the *eleven plus*, the passing of which meant that you were given the opportunity to go to grammar school. I am not going to spend time reflecting on the rights and wrongs of such a decision here, however I am going to make the point that, once again, it was the teachers at that school who saw something in me that they must have recognised as potential.

Looking back now, I would have to say that those years at that school were some of the happiest of my life. It was whilst I was there that I was to go on holiday for the first time ever. The Headteacher became aware of a summer camping trip run by a group of trainee teachers, which was free and I was chosen as someone who qualified. Of course, I did not want to go and by now you, the reader, are all too familiar with the reasons why. Yet when I found out my friends were going, that it was only for five days and that it was not that far away, I was persuaded to go and I was glad I did. Remember that this was a little boy who had never even seen the sea and although we were far from the coast, it was my first taste of fun-filled adventure. We roamed through woods, lit and sang songs around campfires, played games, went on coach trips and enjoyed getting to know the student teachers who appeared to be totally dedicated to making us happy. This, I thought, was what life could be like.

In this part of the book I am trying to inject rays of sunshine into what so far has, perhaps, not been an easy read. Looking back now I am convinced that the school was dedicated not just to educating the children entrusted to their care but making them, as far as possible, feel happy, safe and secure.

I could go on how I remember with fond memories, trips to the zoo, safari park and places of historical interest. There were Christmas parties, fancy dress competitions, discos and for those of us weak in stature, free milk. I played regularly for the football team, delivered milk to classrooms and even became the bell monitor - a very important role as it signalled the start of playtime and the end of the school day. None of this works, of course, without the professionalism, dedication, hard work and perhaps most importantly of all, the care and love of teachers. It is they who made that school, for me, the happy and safe environment I needed and without them I do not honestly know where I would be today. They provided me with the best educational opportunities possible at the time and surrounded that with love. Within that context, I learned that there was another part of me which I hoped one day would thrive.

For this reason I want to end this section with a few words specifically aimed at teachers. *You might never know what a profound effect you have on the lives of young people entrusted to your care. I appreciate just how demanding, difficult and all-consuming your job can be at times but you, literally, have the power to transform lives. For that reason, you have my utmost admiration and respect, not just because of your role as educators because I know the job goes much deeper than that but for every ounce of effort you put in to making the lives of children entrusted to your care better. For this reason, it is hard for me to imagine any teacher not holding before themselves each day what is in the best interests of the children. The emotional energy needed to do this cannot be underestimated and it is a huge responsibility. It requires dedication, commitment, hard work, long hours but above all else, an acute desire to help others realise their potential. None of this, in my opinion, is achievable without caring and dare I say it, loving each and every individual child entrusted to your care. Sometimes, I know, this takes place against the backdrop of extreme social and economic deprivation, making your job even more difficult but all the more important. I, myself, am living proof of what can happen when teachers love a child to the point that it hurts. Yet those teachers, in that school, transformed my life forever. For this reason I want to say a big 'thank you' to them and to all teachers. At times, it may well feel that you are not valued or appreciated but I can assure you of one thing: that for every child whose life you change, whether they can articulate it or not, they will be eternally grateful. So to all those hard-working teachers out there who, day in and day out, do everything they can to make life better for some of the poorest, deprived and most vulnerable children in our society, I salute you. Maybe one day society will both recognise and appreciate what you do but until then, take some comfort from the fact that here, in this book, in these words and in my own way, I pay you the highest tribute I can.*

Finally then, let me go back to that little boy I have told you so much about. I find it amazing, even now when I think back, that the teachers in that school would invest so much time, energy and effort in someone they did not even know. It takes a special kind of person to do that. It takes an even more special kind person to do that simply because they cared. When you are in a dark place, what you need more than anything else is a glimpse of the light, no matter how small, just to let you know that there is hope. For me thinking back, it was like being in a room with no windows and no lights, there was a door but the handle was on the outside and I could not open it by myself. Then along came those teachers and they not only opened the door but also lifted me up and, literally, carried me out into the light. What would have become of me if that never happened is a question I sometimes ask myself. Of course, I cannot answer it with any degree of certainty; all I do know is that I will be eternally grateful for the kindness and love those teachers gave me all those years ago. So if you are a teacher reading this, please never doubt the profound effect you have, every day, on the young people entrusted to your care. You will know far better than me that teaching is not just standing up in front of a class and imparting knowledge but rather, caring for and nurturing the whole person. Of course, some children will need more care than others but very often weak, vulnerable, traumatised and abused young people only have one secure person in their life whom they can turn to in times of crisis and trust, and that is their teacher. In my own life such teachers, in many ways, saved me by helping me find deep within myself someone worth saving. It would take me a long time to rationalise this and work it out but without their help, the danger is that I might have been lost forever and remained a '*Stranger to myself*'.

'Tears For Fears'

This might come as a bit of surprise to some people but I am now going to write something, briefly, about a British pop-rock band formed in Bath, England, in 1981. My intention in this chapter has been, and continues, to be offering rays of light in the darkness so that hope and not despair prevails. Right from the start of my analysis, the title of the band had huge significance for me because in many ways, '**Tears For Fears**' aptly described how I felt and therefore, experienced life. I lived a life of fear, finding expression through silent tears which no one responded to. Later in life, it came as a revelation to me that this pop-rock band were writing songs and music about those things in my life which I have already described in the previous chapter. As a result of this, perhaps, for the first time in my life, I began to realise that other people were going through what I thought was exclusive to me. To discover that you are, in fact, not alone but that others were out there too, sharing their experiences to help those who were suffering; eventually became an integral part of my own healing.

Their first album was called '*The Hurting*' and it was released in 1983. If you get a moment, have a look at the front cover and you will see a small child sitting down sideways on, with his knees drawn up and his little hands covering his face. The album is about childhood trauma and the front cover and the title track make this abundantly clear. As you listen to each song, you are drawn into what I can only describe as a set of experiences which reveal the traumatic life of the child involved. Songs such as '*Pale Shelter*', '*Memories Fade*', '*Suffer the Children*', '*Watch Me Bleed*' and '*Start of the Breakdown*', all reflect on what is going on inside the mind and heart of the child, as the words and music invite the listener into what might be described as a '*Mad World*'. Over and over again it feels like the child is trapped in a set of circumstances beyond his or her control, their life dominated by fear, but their response can only be expressed in tears. Remember that little boy sobbing his heart out at that desk in that school, desperate to be with his mother to keep her safe?

For me, this album is so important because, in my opinion, it successfully encapsulates in both words and music how I felt and what was going on inside of me all those years ago. In all honesty, I have never had the courage to share many of the experiences I have described in the pages of this book with anyone before but the work of '**Tears For Fears**' began to suggest for me that one day, at least, this might just be possible.

Their second album, '***Songs from the Big Chair***', was released in 1985 and saw both a continuation of, and a progression from, '***The Hurting***'. Once again for me, songs like '*I Believe*' and '*Broken*', retained the essence of their previous work, by reflecting on the consequences of childhood trauma. But there was also a noticeable change, in so far as it became clear to me that to stay with such painful memories indefinitely, was potentially harmful. This is where the song '*Shout*' comes in and the need to '*let it all out*' shines a light on the need for help and support from someone else, if the effects of childhood trauma are to be addressed and some form of healing take place. As a result, there appears to be something positive, at last, in the song, '*Head Over Heels*' but notice its direct link to the track '*Broken*' I referred to earlier. The title for the album, '**Songs From The Big Chair**', comes from the 1976 television film '**Sybil**', about a woman with multiple personality disorder who only feels safe when she is sitting in her analyst's '**big chair**'. As a result, the message is clear about the need to give voice to the trauma if any sort of healing is ever going to take place. It would take me a long time, personally, to appreciate just how important this is.

By the time we come to the third and final album I have chosen, '**The Seeds of Love**' released in 1989, things have changed musically and thematically. It is well beyond the scope of this book to reflect on the nature of *consciousness* and what this means for our mental health. Earlier, I used the term '*awareness*' when discussing such concepts because in many ways, for me at least, they mean the same thing. In this album, 'Tears For Fears' explore the need for *self-awareness* if healing is ever going to take place. The opening track, '*Woman in Chains*', sets about this in a complex way, by reflecting on the need for men to acknowledge their feminine side; the suppression of which can lead to all sorts of complex problems. If there is a theme to the whole album, I would have to say it is in identifying the need to *look beyond the self*, not to stay with the trauma of the past but to be reconciled with it and to move outward; however, to achieve this you have to become, *self-aware*. The title track, '*Sowing the Seeds of Love*', encourages a movement outwards beyond the self, whilst '*Standing on the Corner of the Third World*' seeks to promote engagement by the individual with the world outside the self. However, there are also moments of warning as in '*Bad Man's Song*', which highlights and stresses the need not to fall into the trap of seeing the world through the projections others place on you - an issue I explored personally in the earlier part of this book. When we come to '*Advice For The Young at Heart*', we begin to understand that the hard road to recovery is in the past but the key to healing, is to progress from the personal to the social. The key to all of this though is *consciousness* or being *aware* of the issues involved. Hence, **'Swords and Knives'** explores the possible consequences of failing to achieve this whilst **'Year of the Knife'** highlights the great truth; that is to say, the vital importance of achieving *consciousness*, which will, in the end lead to healing.

In the first part of this book I spent a long time exploring my own route to finding *consciousness* or *awareness*. **'Tears For Fears'** do this in a different way but come to the same conclusion, that the key to eventual healing is to discover a reality beyond the self. For this reason, a journey must take place with its ultimate goal being engagement with the world. Yet there is so much preventing us from living real and authentic lives because of the roles we adopt in relation to our expectations of others. This is where we meet *'the stranger'* within and if we are not careful, become him or her and so, as a result, are completely unaware that we are, in fact, not living real lives and therefore, not being our true selves. **'Tears For Fears'** shed light on this whole process and the journey, which must take place from childhood trauma to the liberated self, fully alive and engaged with the world.

Perhaps it is possible to see this as a sort of ascension, which is to say a gradual movement away from internal pain, suffering and the self-doubt it brings to community, which is of course, greater than the individual. There is a song by 'Tears For Fears' on the re-mastered version of 'The Seeds of Love' called 'Always In the past', which reflects on the need not to live in the past but to be always on the move towards a brighter and better future. The aim of this process is what I would call 'wholeness', leading ultimately to a complete recognition and acceptance of the self but within a social and therefore, communal context. If, therefore, I had to make a direct link between the work of 'Tears For Fears' and their 'Seeds of Love' album with my own reflections in the earlier part of this book, I would have to say that both involve a call to 'wake up'! This might be termed 'The Great Truth', which most of us fail to recognise but it enables us to see life as it is, to confront 'the stranger' and most importantly of all, to find the freedom to be our true selves. It takes a tremendous amount of courage to see beyond the self because as the song, 'Standing on the Corner of the Third World' puts it, it is far easier to live life 'like a mussel in a shell'.

The great hope for me in reflecting on the essence of this body of work, was to recognise that progress was possible and although the hard road to recovery was in my past, I did not have to stay there. Yet sometimes you do have to go backwards in order to go forward in life and that both feeling and thinking can go hand in hand to aid recovery. As a result, it still feels strange to me that I could find a resonance between my own experiences of life and what a pop-rock band were exploring and writing about all those years ago. Yet I did and it helped my own self-reflection process, especially when you think that I was doing this all by myself. There comes a moment though, when you consciously realise that you are not the only one feeling the way that you do and, in and of itself, that moment is what I would call, progress.

Once again, I offer these words both as a personal reflection but now also in the hope that anyone who reads them might, in some small way, also be helped. The tenure of the previous chapter was very much in the mould of '*Shout, Shout Let it All Out*' but this chapter, I hope, has moved on to '*Sowing the Seeds of Love*' and that also is progress. So whoever you are and wherever you are, '*Don't give up*'!

'Sticks in the Mud'
CHAPTER NINETEEN

I have an early memory of a little boy all by himself in the front garden of his run down and dilapidated back-to-back council house. High walls surround him and the rest of the world seemed so very far away, almost as if it did not exist. There is cardboard in the bottom of his shoes to keep his feet dry because of the holes, his jumper is threadbare at the elbows and he is wearing odd socks. At the same time, although the weather is cold, damp and wet he is wearing short, grey trousers, perhaps a size or two too big for him. He is on his knees by the side of a rather large puddle, surrounded by soft mud. In his hands are two sticks, one of which he drops gently into the water whilst using the other to push it away. He smiles as he imagines that the stick is a ship, sailing across the sea to where he does not know. Then he has an idea - what if he could gather more sticks and using the mud, make a small fort on the other side of the puddle and then the ship would have somewhere to go. So he stands up and goes in search of his prize. 'This should be fun,' he thinks.

By now you know the context of that little boy's life but here is the thing. Will he remain a chicken or does he have another destiny, to fly like the eagle? People have asked me, 'Why have you written this book and who is it for?' All the way through I have tried to be brutally honest and at times, as I am sure you can imagine, it has not been easy. In many ways I have written this book for myself, to put down on paper the journey I have been on. The process has allowed me to organise my thoughts and reflect deeply on what has happened to me, how such experiences have shaped my life and what they have meant for me as a person. However, it is also true that I have written this book in the hope that somehow by sharing my own experiences of life and how I have made sense out of them; the process might be of some help to others who are also struggling to cope.

Thinking back now, it is tremendously important that the little boy does not stay where he is, playing with his sticks in the mud. However, you now know part of his story and what will happen to him. No one will come to his rescue. The walls I described, surrounding him in that garden, are both real and metaphorical and will keep him where he is. In fact, eventually they will close in on him and crush the very life out of his little body. Yet it is important that we do not fall into a state of despair. I have provided glimpses of hope, rays of light in the darkness, which will eventually bear fruit but he will have to make sense out of it all for himself. This, of course, will come much later but this book is an attempt to outline how such a process is possible, though its success will depend on the individual. There can be no substitute, however, for direct help; a real hand holding yours in the darkness. To know that there is somebody interested in your story, who cares about you and is willing to do whatever it takes to help. Yet going back to my *chicken* and *eagle* analogy, people may well help you, they may not, of course, but it is only you who can make that first leap off the ground. In other words, as I have said repeatedly in the first part of this book, the breakthrough moment for me came when I first became *aware* that not only that I had to do something but that I actually could. That was a moment of supreme liberation. The realisation that I would not allow the walls to crush the life out of me and I could be free to be my true self. The key, however, was appreciating that first leap being only the starting point of my journey because, in truth, I had not learned to fly yet but was merely flexing my wings. So inevitably, I fell back to the ground and it hurt but to have glimpsed some of the possibilities that lay out there was more than worth it. You see, you cannot learn to fly overnight and time and time again you will tumble back to the ground and lie flat on your back but the key is not to stay there. Get up and leap again and again and again until that moment comes when you soar. Then, and only then, can you really afford to look down or look back, but you will do so with a new set of eyes and see things in a completely different way. This, in essence, is a metaphorical summary of this book and hopefully paints a picture of hope.

When I reflected on the music of '**Tears For Fears**' in the last chapter, I suggested a progression of thought across their first three albums from the trauma of the interior world to the liberation of life within a meaningful social and communal context. I referenced this process as one of being a sort of *ascension*. However, I could also use the word *transcendence* to describe that moment when you actually learn to fly, to be one with yourself, to be comfortable with whom you are and to take your rightful place in the world.

I do not think it too strong a thing to say, therefore, that at last you have begun to find meaning in life. Notice here too that I am no longer just talking about myself but am gently offering this out to others, as a possible means to be reconciled with yourself and the world. To this end, there does at some point need to be a shift from self to others in terms of well-being because, it has been my experience that you cannot have one without the other. Think back to my description of the teachers who helped me as a perfect example of where this might lead. Ultimately, I discovered by flying, things about myself which would only make sense within a social or communal context. Let me explain.

In this book, at least in part, I have shared with you some of the story of my life, admittedly most of which, has come from my childhood. This life narrative I identified as me, but eventually I reached the stage of my life when it had to make sense. Thus I could not leave that little boy alone in the mud with his sticks because I needed to do something about it. Hence, I had to go back to those painful memories, some of which I shared with you, and make sense out of them within the broader context of my life story. Only then could any kind of healing take place. If that was the first stage, then the next was to fly higher looking for even deeper meaning, which for me could only be found in and through love. It seems strange to say this but after everything I have said in the pages of this book, I can sum it all up by saying that I needed to learn to love myself. Does that sound easy to you? Try it and see! Even now, all these years later, I still do not find it easy but it is, at least for me, an essential part of the process. What comes next is just as powerful; a sense of belonging and with that, the realisation that you are truly loved because of who you are. I learnt that at school and it was to transform my life forever. In the pages of this book, I have said very little about the power and vital impact of my mother's love on my life, without which I truly do not know what would have become of me. I have written about this elsewhere, so for now I am going to put this to one side but her love rescued me from certain oblivion!

Finally, let me bring things together a little bit because once you how learn to fly, are reconciled with yourself, know that you belong and are loved; all of a sudden your life has a purpose. The process I have described in this book enabled me to recognise my own strengths and weaknesses and to embrace them. Once I could do that, then I was also able to recognise what motivated me, what strengths I had and eventually I could use this to help others. Notice here the process of progression I described earlier and how what I am saying now has both social and communal significance. In other words there has been a shift in emphasis from myself to the other. Would the *'stranger'* have allowed this to happen I wonder? What kind of person would I have been if what I call *'awareness'* had not taken place? As I write these words, I cannot help but conclude that the *'stranger to myself'* I had become, would not have allowed me to do so. In the end, there is a realisation that life can have meaning and purpose, that by being your true self there is the strength to help others, which in turn only serves to confirm that the progression is complete and that after all, I have something worthwhile to do. This book gives tangible expression to my yearning to reach out to others and to say that you are not alone, there are people out there who care about you who love you and will do anything they can to help you. One day you might even discover, like I did, that you are, in fact, that person.

IS THIS THE END OR JUST THE BEGINNING?
CHAPTER TWENTY

It seems such a long time ago when I first sat down to write this book, five years in fact. At first I found myself writing with enthusiasm, drawing heavily on my own experiences of life. Then all of a sudden I would just stop. Sometimes it would be weeks, on other occasions months and even years before I could return to the project. Deep down, however, I knew that it was something that I simply had to complete. Thinking about it now, there were two reasons for this. Firstly, I had to do it for myself because the memories I had, particularly from childhood, had haunted me for too long. Secondly, it dawned on me that, perhaps, others could be helped by what I had been through. These two factors then became my primary motivation for writing but equally, I was also aware of the fact of the sheer number of people that I knew that had, or were suffering from, mental health issues. Society is also now beginning to recognise just how important mental health is but the scale of the problem is huge. I would be the first to admit that I am no psychologist, psychotherapist, counsellor or psychiatrist; in fact, I have no expertise in these areas at all. What I am, though, is a person, a fellow human being who has experienced the trauma, mental anguish and the cruelty of life. In the pages of this book, all I have tried to do is reflect on my own experience and share them with others in the hope that somehow, they might be of some help to someone else.

If you have made it this far you will have noticed a significant difference between the two parts of the book. In Part One, I enter into a conversation, which if you haven't guessed by now is in fact, with myself, on which I invite the reader to eavesdrop. Here I share some of my deepest thoughts about the source of my own unhappiness and I come up with a solution, which is that I had become *'a stranger to myself'*. I called this moment of self-realisation *'awareness'* and the more I became *'aware'*, then the more things began to change. For this reason, I refer to Part One as *'Exorcising the Ghost'*, a term which enabled me to sum up the need to confront the *'stranger to myself'* I had become with the real me. The process I describe was not an easy one because my life and society had taught and encouraged me to be someone else. But who, if given a choice, wants to live their life as another person? For this reason, this *stranger* or this *ghost*, literally had to go. Therefore I refused to stay on the ground. After all, why be a *chicken* when I knew, in fact, that I was an *eagle*?

It is this very message that, ultimately, I wanted to convey to my readers. In other words I was saying, '*If I can learn to fly, then why can't you?*' '*If I can be my real self, discover real, authentic and lived happiness just by being me, then why can't you?*' The style of my writing, I hope, has never been to tell people what to do. As I've said before, this is not one of those self-help books: read this and you'll be okay, all your troubles will disappear. If anybody tells you that then it's a lie, pure and simple. Instead, all I have genuinely tried to say is, '*This is me, this is my story, you might find it helpful or you might not but both are equally okay.*' I am sure that, by now you will have your own opinion on this, which is part of who you are and that's absolutely fine too, but the things I have shared with you about my life in the pages of this book are genuine, honest and sincere and I hope this comes through. For me, the whole process has been hugely demanding and in many ways it still is but the key I found was, as I said in an earlier chapter, learning to *surf* and not sinking beneath the daunting waves of life. Yet I knew I couldn't just leave it there, that I owed it to my readers to go even deeper into my story and share with them, and therefore you, some of my specific experiences of life the most traumatic of which lay in my childhood.

For this reason, the second part of the book adopts a very different style. This is because I wanted to make a contrast between darkness on the one hand and light on the other. As a result I called Part Two, '*The Sun and The Moon*'. Here the moon stands for darkness, unhappiness and despair, whilst the sun represents light, happiness and hope. At the same time both symbolise movement, as the sun appears to move across the sky, eventually giving way to the darkness of the night. For many, the sun also represents masculinity with the moon that of femininity. However, both are needed for wholeness, another important feature of Part Two. So the second part of the book focuses very much on contrasts but is embedded with my own real and personal experiences. I suppose, in many ways, I wanted to invite the reader more into my own personal life and to lay bare the truth both of my own trauma, which eventually was to give rise to the person we first met in Part One. However, I was also conscious of trying to maintain the balance between what was a *'personal reflection'*, with my desire, ultimately, to help others. Equally, I was aware of the need to inject life, happiness, hope and light into the project, hence the symbolism of the sun.

'Rebel – Rebel' is a chapter, which I hope will resonate with people of a certain age, though not exclusively so. My primary objective here was to ground my personal experiences in the real world. Most people, sooner or later, link part of their lives with the music, films and television programmes of their youth, which becomes a sort of backdrop to life. So in this chapter I set to work identifying and linking certain significant experiences of my life with the prevailing popular culture of the time and surprisingly, a pattern began to emerge. There were, of course, ups and downs, highs and lows but also a resonance which helped me make some sort of sense out of how I was feeling at the time. When you are in a dark place, sometimes you need an injection of energy to galvanise you into action and this is what I found in

my own musical past. At last, therefore, in this chapter the sun begins to shine but unfortunately not for long! '*Don't Look Back in Anger*', as I am sure you can imagine, was the most difficult chapter for me to write. As a result, we now find ourselves back in the darkness of the night in the company of the moon. Some people, no doubt, will say to me, '*Why did you write this chapter and why did you feel the need to include it in the book?*' The simple answer to this is because I knew I had to; now let me explain why. I was conscious of the fact that much of what I had written in Part One, whilst immersed totally in my own personal experiences of life, was for the most part not grounded in specifics. Equally, there also comes a moment in the process of writing when you do ask yourself, why are you doing this, what is your goal, your aim and your purpose? Time and time again I have been at pains to make the point that this book is a '*personal reflection on my own mental health*', yet I reached the point whereby I knew it had to be more than that. In some way, it had to reach out to others and offer the hand of help. If I was going to do this with any degree of honesty, integrity and credibility, then I knew I would have to share some of my own personal pain with the reader. After all, where did that person come from that I wrote about in Part One? How was he formed, what had he been through; who was he really? So in *'Don't Look Back in Anger,'* I laid bare some of my most traumatic childhood memories and experiences and invited the reader into my life. Boy was it tough to relive some of those childhood experiences and at times, I just had to stop and walk away from my keyboard because it all became a little too much. Yet I did it for two reasons. Firstly for myself, as I recognised that unless I could be reconciled with my own childhood trauma there could be no healing and secondly, for the reader and, therefore, for anyone who has or is still going through such experiences themselves. However, the chapter ends with a message of hope linked to its title and my belief that in some way we are all traumatised by life but that, in fact, does not have to be the end of our stories because healing and wholeness, for all of us, is always possible.

We now come to one of the most important chapters in the book, *'Don't Give Up'*, and a return to the light of the sun. Eventually, I became conscious of the fact that if healing for me, at least, was ever going to take place, then I could not stay in the past and I could not stay alone with my own thoughts. Hence there had to be a movement outwards from the self to the social or communal. That is to say from my internal life and pain to, that of the external world and engagement with and in it. Yet how was I to do that when my whole life had been consumed by internal suffering? The answer, of course, was that I needed help, which could only come from outside of myself. It was at this point that I recognised the important role certain teachers had in my life and so I set about piecing together and identifying all those teachers, in fact, who had helped me for no other reason other than I needed help. I must say this became a revelation to me, hence that is why I spent so much time not only recounting certain critical moments in my time at school, but why I also was at pains to pay my own tribute to the much underappreciated teaching profession. If I learned anything from this part of the process it was that it is difficult, if not impossible, to achieve any kind of healing or wholeness by yourself. Those teachers taught me an important life lesson; that I could not stay alone in the darkness of my childhood trauma forever because if I did, then in the end, it would result in my own destruction. Instead, I had to come out of the darkness and into the light, note here the sun and moon imagery, and take my rightful place in the world.

This process of movement was confirmed for me when I explored the work of '**Tears For Fears**'. Not only did they write music and songs about childhood trauma but they also emphasised the importance of movement or progression from the inner world to that of the world outside. This is why that to be healthy, our lives must have a social or communal dimension to them. However, the key to this seemed to be something for them which also resonated with me and that was *consciousness*, or what I called in Part One of this book, *awareness*. Only once we have become *aware* of something, *conscious* of it, can we begin to do something about it. This, therefore, in many ways is where Part One of the book meets Part Two and the result is progress. Hence, there now comes a shift in emphasis with the focus now being far more on the sun. Progress is, of course, never easy and not for one minute will I ever say that it is but despite the setbacks, despite the failures, despite the times when we all stumble and fall; we need to pick ourselves up and keep moving towards the light. In other words, '*Don't give up*'!

Finally we come to '*Sticks in the Mud*', where I hope everything comes together. Pain and suffering is common to all of us but it is true that some suffer more than others. It is a sad thing for me to say but even today, many children continue to suffer all kinds of childhood trauma with much of it going on behind closed doors. In the same way, we are now becoming increasingly aware of those who suffered such trauma many years ago and who have still have not been able to come to terms with it. Once again I find myself saying, that is one of the reasons you have written this book - to shed some light on the darkness of childhood trauma. Ultimately, my main motivating factor for writing this book was that I saw myself standing in the midst of a society that was crying silent tears. It was almost as if every person that I met was in some way suffering from some kind of internal anguish. Part of me knew that I could not just stand by and do nothing, the only question I asked myself was, what? Then I remembered that little boy playing with those '*sticks in the mud*' all those years ago. If I could go back to him, I would pick him up, hold him in my arms and offer him a way out and therefore, a better life. That, my friends, ultimately, is the reason why I have written this book. In the hope that it might be of help to someone out there who is alone and crying silent tears in the darkness.

Finally if I could offer, in all humility, one piece of advice to anyone suffering any kind of mental anguish, it would be to seek help from others. You see there are people out there who care about you, people who you can trust and people who will do anything it takes to make your life better. People who will literally dry your silent tears and help you find your way back into the light. Then one day you might realise that you are, in fact, one of those people too.

Good-bye.

Good luck.

Jon

To my sons:

'I hope by now you can see how I knew how you felt and what you were going through all along.'

Dad

Acknowledgements

The publishers and authors would like to thank Russell Spencer, Matt Vidler, Susan Woodard, Janelle Hope Leonard West, Lianne Bailey-Woodward, Laura Jayne Humphrey and Katie Major for their work, without which this book would not have been possible.

About the Publisher

L.R. Price Publications is dedicated to publishing books by unknown authors.

We use a mixture of both traditional and modern publishing options, to bring our authors' words to the wider world.

We print, publish, distribute and market books in a variety of formats including paper and hardback, electronic books, digital audiobooks and online.

If you are an author interested in getting your book published, or a book retailer interested in selling our books, please contact us.

www.lrpricepublications.com

L.R. Price Publications Ltd,

27 Old Gloucester Street,

London, WC1N 3AX.

020 3051 9572

publishing@lrprice.com

Printed in Great Britain
by Amazon

17855414R00119